Fight to Live

WINNING THE SPIRITUAL AND PHYSICAL BATTLE FOR YOUR HEALTH

KRISTY DOTSON
CHRISTINE TENNON

Fight to Live : Winning the Spiritual and Physical Battle for Your Health
by Kristy Dotson & Christine Tennon

Published by: KINGDOM COME, LLC
                 www.FightingToLive.com

Library of Congress Control Number: 2007903997

07 08 09 10 11 12 13   9 8 7 6 5 4 3 2 1
Printed in the United States of America

It is with great honor that we dedicate this book to:

Pastor Bill Winston
Living Word Christian Center
Forest Park, Illinois

Thank you, Pastor Winston, for teaching us to pursue our God-ordained mission each day with faith and fortitude. Not only do you teach but you also demonstrate an active faith that produces much fruit. We strive to do likewise as the Holy Spirit leads. Out of this determination, *Fight to Live* was birthed. May it edify the body of Christ and bring honor to our Lord's holy name.

Kristy Dotson & Christine Tennon

Kristy Dotson & Christine Tennon

Table of Contents

Introduction.. 7

Part One: Spiritual Warfare

Chapter One 13
Destinies Derailed

Chapter Two... 27
Understanding the Battle

Chapter Three.. 41
Abandoned Authority

Chapter Four 51
Does It Really Run in the Family?

Chapter Five... 65
Surrounded by the Enemy

Chapter Six... 77
The Motive Behind the Meal

Chapter Seven 85
Love and War

Chapter Eight 93
Feast or Fast?

Chapter Nine 103
Denying Yourself

Chapter Ten.. 115
Lessons from the Tabernacle

Part Two: Physical Warfare

Chapter Eleven.. 129
Boot Camp

Chapter Twelve.. 137
Counting the Costs

Chapter Thirteen 153
Weapons of Warfare

Chapter Fourteen.. 169
Casualties of War

Chapter Fifteen.. 185
Filthy Lucre

Chapter Sixteen.. 191
Magic Bullets

Chapter Seventeen 201
Kingdom Nutrition

Chapter Eighteen.. 221
Pay Now or Pay Later

Chapter Nineteen 237
Severed Supplies

Chapter Twenty.. 247
Faith Without Works

Chapter Twenty-One... 259
Amazing Grace

Chapter Twenty-Two 271
Sweet Surrender

Nutritional Education Resources 279

Additional Resources 281

Introduction

STOP! This book comes with a warning. Don't worry — its content is not sexual or violent. But it does address a subject few people ever want to discuss. Here goes ...

Are you consistently handling your health and nutrition in a way that is pleasing to God? Maybe these are some of the ways you'd answer this question:

"Well, the Lord knows my heart is willing but my flesh is weak."

"I'm only human and can only do so much."

"I figure if God made it, I can eat it. After all, I have to have some fun!"

These are natural responses to a supernatural problem. What's the problem? Too much sickness and disease caused by things we can control, such as our diets and the amount of exercise we get. This problem is not only interfering with the quality of our day-to-day lives but also with the work to be done for the kingdom of God. It is a curse set in motion by Satan in the Garden of Eden and now it's time to reverse it. Now is the time to make the connection between diet, exercise, and destiny. Now is the time to take back stolen territory that lands too many of God's children in the hospital or the graveyard before they finish their divine assignments. Now is the time to exercise authority over our health.

So drop that Twinkie and get ready to make some decisions — and act on them!

First, stop worshiping couch potato lifestyles and dead foods. You know what they are. They're the stuff strategically placed in the middle aisles of the grocery store with ingredients we cannot pronounce. Much of the menu items at many fast food joints. The super-sized servings at popular chain restaurants, fried in partially hydrogenated oil and smothered in salt. The sweet treats prepared with four to five different sugars that seem to find us wherever we go. The "snacks" crowding our kitchen cabinets and crying out to us as we sit for hours in front of the television or late at night when we are bored or depressed.

These foods have become our sacred cows, even in the body of Christ. People are bowing at the table not just to say grace but also to pay homage to a variety of killer foods put before them. Meanwhile, the objects of our passion at mealtime are too often our poison. So if this topic is a No Trespassing zone for you, prepare to have your boundaries breached!

At this point, you may be thinking, *Oh, great. Just what the world needs, another book on how to diet or lose weight.* WRONG! That is not the message of this book. It is about the "why" — a "why" that does not get much attention. *Why* this struggle is more spiritual than natural. *Why* spiritual warfare against those who push killer foods is uncharted territory. *Why* Satan's role in our food-related healthcare crisis is under exposed. *Why* Christians must raise up an organized standard against this assault. And *why* good health must be a priority for believers who want to finish the work God has assigned them. This is a consciousness-raising message designed to help you keep Satan under your feet at breakfast, lunch, snack time, and dinner. Since Satan wants you dead, you must immediately — once and for all — make up your mind to stop helping him kill you!

As with everything else in life, there is a spiritual perspective and a worldly point of view. Food consumption is no exception. There are powers in the unseen realm constantly trying to influence our lifestyles so we will destroy ourselves. What better weapon than food? We need it to live, right? It is one of life's simple pleasures, is it not? What's wrong with indulging a little? After all, we have to have some enjoyment, don't we? True. All true. But we can destroy ourselves by not controlling this "enjoyment."

Self-control is still a fruit of the spirit. This is in stark contrast to a world that promotes a "see it, want it, eat it" mentality. Saying no is almost considered abnormal. In fact, people will even challenge you when you try to restrain yourself at mealtime. But with any war, you must know who is for you and who is against you in order to win the fight. So if you are ready to see how your perspective on food and fitness lines up with the Word of God, read on. But be warned again. This is not a "how to" book. It has no recipes or step-by-step instructions on how to eat or lose weight. There is more than enough information in the marketplace on that subject. But if you are looking to dig deeper, to understand "why" staying healthy seems to be such a struggle, even for Christians, then keep reading.

"Healthcare crisis" is now a common phrase in our American vocabulary. Everybody knows or should know we are in one. But look at the situation from God's point of view. Compare what he says about managing your health to how you actually manage it. Bottom line: if your current diet does not line up with biblical teachings on physical wellness, you should not change your diet until you first change your mind about what food does for you and against you.

You may think, *I eat a pretty healthy diet. I only go out to restaurants two to three times a week and I try to get in some vegetables once or twice a week; I am doing okay.* But look around. Health and fitness is a multi-billion dollar industry. Yet we are getting fatter and sicker every day. The dollars are being spent but the results are disastrous. It does not take a Rhodes scholar to figure out something is terribly wrong.

Everyone from actress Suzanne Somers to TV psychologist Dr. Phil McGraw, and every kind of new age guru in between, is telling us how to lose weight. We have fitness centers in virtually every neighborhood, workout specials at the local YMCA, diet pills, diet food, Weight Watchers, Jenny Craig, Pilates, aerobics, workout videos, toning balls, treadmills, exercise bikes, Stairmasters, running clubs, fat-free candy, sugar-free candy, Slim-Fast, the Atkins diet, the South Beach diet, the grapefruit diet, liquid diets, thousands of vitamins and supplements and a gazillion other gadgets on the market to supposedly "help" us stay healthy. Yet people in increasing numbers are still dying from diseases caused by obesity and nutritional deficits — including those claiming Jesus Christ (the Great Physician) as Savior.

As believers, we have a responsibility to show the world a better way. Needless to say, we are long overdue for circling the wagons in this war for good health. Thousands of Christians — and many others for that matter — are being slain daily on this battlefield. From a physical standpoint, believers look like the world in terms of our physical conditions and we too often die from the world's diseases. This is not God's plan for his holy nation — the royal priesthood redeemed by the blood of Christ for good works on earth. So the time has come to take authority over this situation and begin living and looking like the King's kids. The only way to do this is to treat this situation like the war it clearly is.

Part One

Spiritual Warfare

Kristy Dotson & Christine Tennon

Chapter One

Destinies Derailed

For we are God's [own] handiwork (His workmanship), recreated in Christ Jesus, [born anew] that we may do those good works, which God predestined (planned beforehand) for us [taking paths which He prepared ahead of time], that we should walk in them [living the good life which He prearranged and made ready for us to live].
~ Ephesians 2:10 (AMP)

"Karen is in heaven. She died at 5:49 p.m. on Friday. She left a wonderful legacy."

I (Kristy) heard these words on my voicemail Saturday, April 16, 2005, after I returned home from a full day of appointments and checked my messages. This one was flagged "urgent" and I knew before I listened to it that what I was about to hear would not be good. Sure enough, my brother-in-law's voice delivered the sobering news that my oldest sister, Karen, had lost the battle of her life at age fifty-two because of a negative reaction to a pharmaceutical drug. In disbelief, I pressed the replay key on my telephone, hoping perhaps I had misunderstood the message. Unfortunately, I had heard correctly. My sister was gone.

Looking back on that day, I remember vividly my initial reaction and the wide range of emotions that followed. First, sadness overtook me. This was my big sister, my role model, my mentor. How could she be taken away at the drop of a hat? She was too nice, too sweet, too caring. She was one who had figured out what she was born to do and was in the process of fulfilling her God-given assignment. Everyone loved her presence and demeanor. How could Satan take her? How could she abandon *me* in this cruel, confusing world? She had two kids and a wonderful husband. How could she possibly leave *them*?

My sadness immediately turned into anger. "Satan, I am sick of you!" I cried out in despair. "One by one you keep taking the lives of so many people, and you have convinced the masses your activities are normal and acceptable as a part of life!" And now the death angel had robbed me of my sister. I was fed up! Fed up with people dying due to sickness and disease! Fed up with an enemy that had gone too far this time!

Wiping away my tears, I suddenly felt the urge to pull out an old photo album that contained pictures of my sister. I had to see her face and somehow mentally accept the fact that she had physically left this earthly realm. My mind could not accept this truth as reality. I guess this was because just the week before when she was in the hospital fighting for her life, seeing her walk in wholeness again was all I could think. My prayer and confessions had focused only on the positive and not on the negative.

There had not been one ounce of doubt in my heart that she would be healed and that the manifestation of her healing was imminent. The precious blood of Jesus had already purchased it. As she lay in the hospital, I received reports that her kidneys and liver had shut down and that she was on life support, but my faith remained unwavering. I had joined forces with an army of other believers who matched their faith with mine and stood in the gap on Karen's behalf. So when I received the unfortunate news, my spirit literally rejected the report.

I thumbed through my family album and reminisced over past events and outings shared with my sister. Uncontrollable tears rolled down my face by the bucket-load. There were pictures of my parent's fiftieth wedding anniversary, business conventions I had attended, and shots of my vacations at her home in Las Vegas. As I flipped from page to page, only one thought came to mind. As this truth rolled over and over in my head, I formed the words to articulate it and finally just had to shout it out:

"She wasn't done living yet! Her assignment on this earth was not complete!"

That was all I could think.

At fifty-two, my sister had not lived out all God had in store for her. What about all the people she was supposed to touch? What about the unsaved to whom she was supposed to minister? What about all the business travel and support she was supposed to offer to her husband? What about her two children whom she had faithfully home-schooled for over twelve years? Who was going to teach them now? *Karen, you left too soon! You were not done living yet!*

A week after my sister's death, I received a call from a friend who knew Karen and me. She expressed her sympathy and then tried to comfort me by saying my sister had lived her life and God had "called her home." As much as I appreciated the phone call, I felt obligated to correct years of false teaching this friend apparently had accepted. My response to her was, "God does not take our lives and call us home. Satan does. If God wanted me dead, he has the power to take me out of here tomorrow. Instead, his mercy grants me another day to fulfill my purpose on earth." With that, the call ended abruptly.

How many of you have had a "Karen" in your life? Someone you knew who was destined for greatness, yet did not live long enough to fulfill his or her dreams and God-given assignments. Someone whose life-breath was snuffed out prematurely by sickness or disease. We see their lives summed up in loving and heart-wrenching words every day in newspaper obituary sections: "Hayden, 44, esteemed lawyer, died of cancer of the stomach and esophagus. He is survived by a wife and two daughters." ... "Cassandra, 57, died of heart failure while awaiting a liver transplant." ... "Jeffrey, 58, dearest husband, died after a long battle with brain cancer." ... "Tracie, 56, former law school dean, died of heart failure." ... "Gerald, 56, died of a heart attack; "great loss" to insurance industry." ... "Anita, 66, a noted cancer researcher, died of gastric cancer at her home." ... "Alex, 5, lost his three-year battle with a brain tumor." ... "Franklin, beloved husband of Melissa, passed away after a courageous battle with stomach cancer." ... "Nolan, charismatic corporate executive, died after a heart attack." ... "Bertha, beloved daughter, passed away from complications of lung disease." ... "Mardine, loving mother, passed away after a long battle with cancer." ... "Jessica, dear wife of Chester, fond sister of Erica." ... "McKenzie, patient, loyal and loving father of Kassie, Sandra, and Arthur." ... "Clarence, beloved husband of Jeraldine, loving father of Kendra." ... "Victoria, a blessing to all who knew her." ... "Linda, a talented equestrian."

On and on it goes. Millions die before their time. Disease or some kind of abnormal health condition sweeps in. Their life potential is reduced to a body in a coffin or ashes in an urn. Their family and friends are left to grieve the loss of life, love, and unfinished dreams. In anguish, many ask, "Why? Why did this happen?"

We have all heard the rather pat answers to this question. They seem to come straight out of a manual on what to say when someone dies. People say things like:

"Well, you know that disease she had runs in her family."

"They did not follow the doctor's orders."

"They should have stuck with the chemo."

"These things just happen."

"It was just their time to go."

And finally, perhaps one of the most frequent responses: "God just took them."

But let's ask some deeper questions about death by disease or a poor health condition and look for some better answers. We might ask:

"How did their cells become cancerous?"

"How did their blood pressure get so high?"

"How did their blood sugar rise to deadly levels?"

"How did their arteries get clogged to the point that blood could not get to their heart or brain?"

"How did the condition that killed them inch its way into their bodies in the first place?"

"How did it get to a point where it ripped them apart bit by bit and finally stopped their breath forever?"

Since blaming God seems to be the popular response, let's look at it from his perspective. God created male and female in his own image. He blessed them and gave them dominion over the whole earth. He told them to be fruitful and multiply (Genesis 1–2). He also prepared work for them to do before they were even born (Ephesians 2:10). His plan was for people to live abundantly (John 10:10) and productively forever in an earthly paradise.

So put aside what the world and some misinformed Christians believe. God does not want to destroy his own creation or just shrug his shoulders when we get sick. He does not look down on earth, see a twenty-four-year-old and label him or her a cancer victim so he can "pluck a flower for his garden." God is love (1 John 4:16) and his desire is that we "prosper in all things and be in health" (3 John 1:2). If God is into plucking us off the planet through sickness and disease, why did Jesus raise Lazarus (see John 11:1-44) and Jairus's daughter from the dead? (See Mark 5:22-24, 35-42.) Why did he heal countless people?

God is not schizophrenic. He would not work against disease on the one hand and then support it on the other. No. Sickness is not part of God's plan for us. But it is part of Satan's plan. Yes. Satan. Lucifer, Beelzebub, that old serpent. Sickness, disease, poverty, addictions, broken homes, broken hearts, broken relationships, crime, misery, natural disasters, plagues, etc., are the tools of his trade. These things came into the world not by the hand of God but by the hand of man and woman who were manipulated by the devil. Adam and Eve set off this chain of calamity when they ate the wrong food at Satan's suggestion and opened the door to worldwide sin. To put things right again, Jesus took on human flesh so that "through death He might destroy him who *had* the power of death, that is, the devil" Hebrews 2:14. (Emphasis added).

Does this mean we are not supposed to die now that Jesus has finished his redemptive work? No. There is "a time to die" (Ecclesiastes 3:2). But we should go from this life to the next God's way. Death by sickness or disease is not his way. It is Satan's. As Chicago-area pastor Bill Winston has often said, *we* should set the appointment to die — not the devil.

Setting an appointment is about exercising authority. According to Hebrews 9:27, "It is appointed for men to die once, but after this the judgment." One of the definitions of *appoint* in *Webster's Dictionary* is "to arrange." A person who arranges an event is in charge and has power to make plans and issue orders. So unless you are a believer who is alive when the Lord returns and are caught up to meet him in the air (see 1 Thessalonians 4:17), you will eventually die or cease to exist in your current physical body. However, your departure should *not* be like those described at the beginning of this chapter. It should be more like the death of Abraham described in Genesis 25:7-8:

> **This is the sum of the years of Abraham's life which he lived: one hundred and seventy-five years. Then Abraham breathed his last and died in a good old age, an old man and full of years, and was gathered to his people.**

And indeed his years were "full." His purpose on earth was mission critical. He was responsible for starting a nation that would serve only the one true God. He finished the job, laid down, and went to be with the Lord. Here was a man who was not even introduced to God until he was seventy-five years old (Genesis 12:1-4). When God told him to leave his home, he obeyed and headed to an unknown place. He acquired great wealth and many servants (Genesis 13:3,7), was envied and yet respected by his neighbors (Genesis 21:22, 23:1-11), led an army against warring tribes to rescue his nephew Lot (Genesis 14), and was an indulgent husband to his beloved, Sarah (Genesis 16). But most importantly, Abraham was the man through whom all the nations of the earth have been blessed. God used him at the ripe old age of one hundred to have a son, Isaac, with his ninety-year-old wife (Genesis 17:17). Through this lineage Jesus Christ was born (Genesis 22:15-18; Matthew 1:1-17).

Sarah lived 127 years (Genesis 23:1). Her assignment was to bear the child God promised to give her and Abraham. Abraham was 137 when she died. But God was not finished with him yet. He took another wife and had six more children with her (Genesis 25:1-2). Truly, Abraham was a man with a very important assignment that took faith *and* flesh — in other words, a physically fit body — to finish. He used the last one hundred of his 175 years on earth to do what God told him to do and then transitioned quietly to the next phase, his eternal life.

Abraham's son Isaac went in a similar fashion. He died at 180 (Genesis 35:28-29) after a full and prosperous life, walking faithfully in God's promises. Isaac's son Jacob got off to a rocky start in life after he stole his brother's birthright. When Jacob met Pharaoh, at the age of 130, he even complained his years had been "few" and not as many as his ancestors (Genesis 47:9). Nevertheless, Jacob fulfilled his God-given purpose in life. He produced the twelve tribes of Israel and died when he was 147 years old (Genesis 47:28). The Bible says when the time for Jacob to die drew near, someone told his son Joseph he was "sick" (Genesis 48:1). Jacob's eyes were "dim with age" (Genesis 48:10). Joseph went to him and Jacob (a.k.a. Israel) "strengthened himself," sat up on the bed (Genesis 48:2) and blessed Joseph's two sons (Genesis 48:9-20).

Jacob then called a meeting with the rest of his sons to tell them what would befall them in the last days. "And when Jacob had finished commanding his sons, he drew his feet up into the bed and breathed his last, and was gathered to his people" (Genesis 49:33). Although it is reported in Genesis 48:1 that Jacob was sick, he was apparently in control of his mind and body. The Bible does not mention that he had any disease. It seems the man was just old and knew it was time to go. Nevertheless, he was able to sit up by himself and draw his feet up into the bed. He had finished his course and had done what God instructed him to do, and went peacefully to meet his maker.

Centuries later, along came Moses. Moses survived the Egyptian infanticide against all natural odds and became the man who led the Israelites out of over four hundred years of slavery. He was forty years old when he fled Egypt to avoid execution for murder. During the next forty years, he shepherded sheep in the Midian wilderness. At that time, the Angel of the Lord appeared to him in a burning bush (Exodus 3:1-10) and told him to return to Egypt and bring the children of Israel out of that land. He was eighty when he told Pharaoh to let the Hebrews go (Exodus 7:7).

What if Moses had succumbed to heart disease at age forty-five? He would have died in the desert, tending sheep. He would have missed the burning bush introduction to God. He would not have lived long enough to return to Egypt and free his Hebrew kinsmen from slavery. He would not have been God's mouthpiece before an arrogant and depraved Pharaoh. He would not have been the instrument through whom God worked mighty miracles and brought down what was at that time the most powerful nation on earth. He would not have been the man to deliver God's law to the Jews — moral codes that to this day influence the content of our modern legislation.

Yes, God had an important job for Moses to do and Moses had the physical strength to carry it out. He was still climbing mountains when he was 120 years old (Deuteronomy

32:48-50) and when he died at that age, "his eyes were not dim nor his natural vigor diminished" (Deuteronomy 34:7). But we don't have to go back centuries to find examples of saints who lived out a good number of years doing God's will, finished their course, and decided when to depart this life.

Steiner A. Dotson, my grandmother, was ninety-seven years old when she passed in 2003. She confessed her salvation at an early age and spent most of her adult years working in ministry. When I (Kristy) was a young child, my grandmother often amazed me, as she was the kind of woman I thought could do anything. She lived alone in a modest country house outside of Montgomery, Alabama. She was the kind of woman who would take you fishing, come home and cook, clean, take a plate of food to a needy family, get ready for church, pick up three fellow members who needed a ride to evening service, attend church, drop off her passengers, and get home around eleven p.m. without muttering a single complaint.

Steiner A. Dotson always seemed to have a peace about her that was a mystery to me until I came to know the Lord. As I grew in Christ, I came to understand the inner peace that stayed with my grandmother day after day after day. I relished the fact that she was ninety-seven years old when she passed. But most of all, I am pleased that my grandmother did not die of cancer, diabetes, stroke, or other maladies that commonly take our elderly loved ones to the grave. Steiner A. Dotson released her soul on October 14, 2003, merely by choosing to "give up the ghost."

I (Kristy) sat at the funeral, basking in the fact that my grandmother had lived well beyond what the world considers an average lifespan. Therefore, her funeral was a day of celebration — not sorrow. Her transition was similar to Abraham's. She enjoyed her life fully, and when she was ready she *chose* the day, the time, and the place. Death did not choose her prematurely. That's because Steiner A. Dotson set the course for her life when she made two critical choices early on. First, she chose Christ and put feet to her faith. Second, she chose good health and took dominion over her flesh when it came to her diet.

So, barring accidents, how long should we expect to live in our present physical form? Before the flood recorded in Genesis 6–7, people lived a long, long time! Adam died after 930 years (Genesis 5:5). Many of his descendants noted in that chapter lived between 800-plus to over 900 years! Enoch did not die at all. The Bible says he "walked with God; and he was not, for God took him" when he was 365 years old (Genesis 5:23-24). This suggests he was there one moment and gone the next, but not because of sickness. Then there's Methuselah, the ever-popular king of longevity who lived 969 years!

At some point before the flood of Noah's day, God shortened humanity's lifespan, saying, "My Spirit shall not strive with man forever, for he is indeed flesh; yet his days shall be one hundred and twenty years" (Genesis 6:3). People were so corrupt and the earth was filled with so much violence during this time that God said he was even sorry he had made man. His heart was grieved and he said he would destroy man to stop the madness. But Noah found grace in God's eyes. He and his immediate family were saved from the floodwaters that destroyed all other humans (Genesis 6:5-22).

In an effort to minimize wickedness, God simply shortened our years after the flood so those who chose to side with Satan would not have hundreds of years to do their evil deeds. This shortened lifespan does not mean God intends for us to die at 120 years of age ravaged by cancer or other horrible diseases. Abraham, Isaac, and Jacob did not go out that way. They even got a few extra years before they slipped into eternity at a time of their own choosing.

However, some people believe the normal human life span is limited to about seventy to eighty years. They base this on a prayer of Moses in Psalm 90. In verse 10, Moses says, "The days of our lives are seventy years; and if by reason of strength they are eighty years, yet their boast is only labor and sorrow; for it is soon cut off, and we fly away." This does not refer to a general lifespan for everyone. It refers specifically to the Israelites, who were afraid to go into the Promised Land because of the giants. These folks complained against God, saying, "If only we had died in the land of Egypt! Or if only we had died in this wilderness!" (Numbers 14:2). The Lord replied, "Just as you have spoken in My hearing, so I will do to you" (Numbers 14:28).

The words out of their own mouths aborted their destinies and they got what they asked for: death in the wilderness. These complaining Hebrews let Satan trick them into believing the life they were living was as good as it was ever going to get, that life in the desert was all they should expect. They did not understand their mission. And they did not understand their God.

Instead, out of fear they chose to die in the wilderness without entering the place of abundance to which God was sending them to set up a powerful kingdom. Their choice did not line up with God's will for them but he loved them enough to let them choose. So they got what they believed and died early at seventy or eighty years. As the Psalm 90 passage above describes, it was a life of labor, sorrow, and eventually a premature death.

Joshua, on the other hand, was an Israelite who trusted God to give the Jews the Promised Land. He did not die in the wilderness. He took the remaining Hebrews into

Canaan after Moses died, led them in many battles against their enemies, and lived to 110 years of age.

Clearly it is not God's will for us to leave this earth at a young or even middle age, or by sickness and disease. If we are living out his purpose, the longer we are here the better it is for the kingdom of God. According to 2 Timothy 1:9, God "has saved us and called us with a holy calling, not according to our works, but according to His own purpose and grace which was given to us in Christ Jesus before time began." God explained this to Jeremiah this way: "Before I formed you in the womb I knew you; before you were born I sanctified you; I ordained you a prophet to the nations." (Jeremiah 1:5). We are no different than Jeremiah. God designed work for us to do even before our natural parents knew we were coming.

Anyone who dies before completing this work and who does not arrange a transition to the next life the way Abraham, Isaac, Jacob, Moses, Joshua, and Steiner A. Dotson did is a victim of destiny thieves. They are the same spirits that struck fear in the Hebrews and tricked them into forfeiting their future in the Promised Land. When it comes to health, these spirits use ignorance, temptation, and popular culture to manipulate people into eating themselves to death. These thieves are not just after your body but your mission as well. And what better tools to use than sickness and disease brought on by poor eating habits? It's a twisted tactic that gets victims to voluntarily consume the poison that kills them.

This is nothing more than dietary terrorism. And it goes about on earth largely unchecked. Our culture continuously feeds this death machine. People and industry drive it, from food manufacturers that *design* food rather than grow it to families who will not take the time to prepare healthy meals, and from drug companies making millions selling magic pills that mask rather than cure sickness to insurance companies that will pay $30,000 for stomach-stapling surgery but won't pay $1,200 for a treadmill. All these things — and then some — converge to create the wave of destruction known as our "health care crisis."

This is not God's plan. When he created the earth, he did not intend for food to be used as a weapon of mass destruction. He made it to keep us alive and well for his purposes. Today, food is manipulated to the point that it is more likely to destroy than preserve or heal a body. Every time a life is taken by killer foods, a divine mission is also taken. And even though many of us know better, we do not do better in this area of life. We simply do not make the connection between what we eat and what we are able to do for God. As evangelist Jesse Duplantis once said during a televised sermon, "Purpose will not permit fleshly indulgence to remove the bloom from spiritual life."

It is long past time for the body of Christ to recommit to good health in order to carry out kingdom assignments. So decide now to keep yourself prepared spiritually, mentally, and physically. For your ears may be assigned to heed the cries for help from around the globe. God may focus your eyes on the weak and downtrodden in your neighborhood or faraway lands. Your hands may be needed to attend the sick and serve the forsaken. Your voice may be commissioned to declare the gospel to the brokenhearted. Your feet may be sent to walk the mission fields as Christ's ambassador to the earth. Your arms may be used to embrace love-starved orphans. Your smile will be needed to bring hope to the hopeless. Yes, you, a member of "a chosen generation, a royal priesthood, a holy nation" (1 Peter 2:9). You are God's own special creation who has a special role to play on the world stage during your appointed season. Plan now to perform it with vigor and finish it in victory! If you don't know what God put you on earth to do, ask him. You might consider praying this prayer:

> **Dear Lord, thank you for being a loving and caring Father. I am grateful to you for caring so much for me that you have given me a purpose in life and provided every resource to ensure your perfect will for me is fulfilled. I put aside my own thoughts and desires and submit to your authority and the order of events you have planned for my time here on earth. Reveal them to me, O Lord, and I will roll all my works upon you, committing and trusting them wholly to you. I pray that each and every day you will cause my thoughts and actions to be aligned with your will, including how I care for my physical body. May everything I do advance your purpose on earth. Thank you, Father, for choosing me and for showing me my part in the big picture. In the name of Jesus I pray. Amen.**

Stories from the Front Lines...

A Missionary's Mission Cut Short by Sickness

In 1990, Cynthia, her husband, and two children went to Brazil as missionaries. They live on the Amazon River, three degrees south of the equator. Cynthia teaches at a missionary school. She describes the climate as very humid with lots of mold and no air conditioning.

Cynthia says, "I haven't always had the best diet. In Brazil, everything we cook is from scratch. We have salad every day consisting of cabbage, tomatoes, carrots, cucumbers, bell peppers, and onions. Periodically we get broccoli and cauliflower and potatoes. A lot rice, potatoes, meat (hamburger, pork, fish). Every morning, the kids break at 10:15 and have snacks, and every day after school they have snacks. Snacks are always sugar snacks, brownies, and cookies. Brazil is really into sugar. I really like to bake and like to make lots of sweets."

While in Brazil, Cynthia became ill with *Candida albicans*, a yeast-related nutritional disorder. She says, "It was hard for me to function every day. Some days I could barely get done what needed to be done. Home would go downhill. All I could do was get to my class and get it done. It also hindered our mission relationships because when I was not feeling well I could not get out and fellowship with those around me, so relationships can dwindle. You're not able to give your all if you are not healthy. There are lots people in our field who are not healthy ... a lot of missionaries."

Messianic Jewish Leader Dies of Cancer

Author, lecturer, and television host Zola Levitt died April 19, 2006 after a valiant fight against cancer. Levitt was a Messianic Jewish believer who accepted Yeshua (Jesus) as Savior in 1971. He was best known for his weekly television program "Zola Levitt Presents" and for his tours of Israel and other parts of the Middle East.

In late March 2006, Levitt wrote a letter about his condition, including the following excerpt that was posted on his website at www.zolalevitt.com:

The Lord has not changed His assignment for me, and so every few days when I feel like I'm having a good

morning, I call together our local film crew and I make another program. Of course, we only broadcast once a week with original programs, so there will be an illusion that I'm pretty well able to do this work, and for now I am. But know four programs will take a month to air, and eight will take two months, and so my condition will undoubtedly deteriorate off-camera. But, on the whole, it's tolerable for now. My orders have not changed. I'm still a soldier manning a post, and my Commander knows I'm wounded.

So, I'll continue this work as long as possible. I think we will probably show some very good repeat performances from the past, and possibly some interview programs while I can do that.

I have the feeling my new orders are coming down, which are that I can start to leave this post, but it will be under protest. I still have one more TV program in mind. And after that I suppose that will be my trip to heaven.

Know that each program I make costs many thousands of dollars, but I like the idea that people see that even a wounded soldier remains useful in the ongoing battle.

Levitt held music degrees from Duquesne University and Indiana University (doctoral coursework completed), and an honorary Doctor of Theology from Faith Bible College. He played the oboe, English horn, recorder, and piano.

Gospel Music Pastor Dies

A seventy-five-year-old pastor died of a stroke after forty years in ministry. She was especially gifted in gospel music and devoted her life to continuous learning, earning five degrees (nursing, psychology, music, religious studies and a doctorate of divinity). This pastor was also active in community affairs.

Chapter Summary

1. God's children are dying prematurely from sickness and disease, contrary to his plan for our lives.
2. More and more people are getting sick or dying before they come to know or fulfill their divine purposes.
3. Satan uses sickness and disease to destroy lives and undermine work that advances the kingdom of God.
4. Christians must wake up to the challenge and overcome it for the sake of fulfilling God's kingdom purposes.

Chapter Two

Understanding the Battle

One of the constants of history is that a nation rarely goes to war until it has convinced itself that victory is attainable and worth the cost. ~ James F. Dunnigan, How to Make War: A Comprehensive Guide to Modern Warfare

Now that you know your purpose or have asked God to reveal it, you need to take a cold, hard look at the current healthcare crisis and how it can destroy your destiny if you don't stay on the alert. Imagine this ...

Scene: *War room in hell. Satan has called a meeting of his top generals and warfare advisors.*

Satan: This meeting of the Council for the Annihilation of Mankind in the area of health and nutrition is now in session. I want reports from all factions assigned to the various industries and organizations that impact the human physical condition: Food, Fitness, Recreation, and Healthcare. We'll start with the food industry.

General Junk Food: I have great news to report! We have just opened up five thousand new hamburger restaurants, each within a one-mile radius of an elementary school. The grand opening featured a two-for-one special on a cheeseburger, fries, and soft drink combo.

In addition, several new products have been introduced into the marketplace. The packaging and advertising are ingenious. One item is a new breakfast bar. It is marketed as a "high energy bar with 50 percent more fiber and 50 percent less sugar." Fortunately, the federal agency responsible for oversight of such matters approved the new sweetener "Slimcose" and agreed to classify it as a vitamin instead of a sugar. It will pack a real wallop when eaten — especially in diabetics. The cravings will be greater than those generated by cookies and candy. And last week we introduced the super-sized version.

We should be able to take out millions of children with this product alone. They were so excited to see it on the market. We threw in a toy to attract the kids and make the parents think they're getting more for their money. With all the hoopla over health these days, we had to come up with something to make people think they're eating healthy while we continue our campaign to have them kill themselves. I'm very pleased with the results so far. Kids are getting fatter by the day. At this rate, they'll get sick a lot faster than their parents. We can eliminate an entire generation with this stuff long before they figure it out and well in advance of them doing anything "good" on earth.

General Fitcon: We have just invented a new gadget to convince people they can lose weight while sleeping. You actually have them attach electrodes to their stomach and plug the unit into the nearest outlet! The advertising campaign is terrific! We've hired some celebrities as spokespeople for this product. It guarantees weight loss of at least thirty pounds in ten days all for just three easy payments of $19.99. The electrodes dry out the skin and can cause a terrible rash in some folks that's almost like a skin cancer. That'll generate a lot of new business for the MDs.

We also have a new weight loss chewing gum on the market. It's filled with toxins that slowly destroy cells. Who knows, it might even cause a new form of cancer for people to throw money at! This gum reduces cravings for sweets but increases the appetite for fried foods. The sweetener is not cane sugar but it's an extract from a South American plant that in the body turns into a product similar to embalming fluid. So by the time the product kills the people who chew it, the undertaker won't have to use as many products to prepare the body for burial!

But the undertaker still can make extra money by offering the family a fancier casket for burying the loved one. It's guaranteed to preserve remains longer after they're in the ground — a full two weeks longer — for just $2,000 more! How's that for a double whammy? Take out the family breadwinner and take the bread, too!

Oops, I'm sorry! I know creating poverty is not my area but I just got carried away. It's all so exciting!

General Give 'Em a Reason to Eat: I have great news, too, commander. My team has just created a new hors d'oeuvres platter that is perfect for all social gatherings such as Super Bowl Sunday, office parties, children's birthday parties, bridal showers, and holiday feasts. It's great for the perfect host or hostess who can serve up a tasty morsel that's cheap and only takes sixty seconds to heat in the microwave. This product looks like a mini potpie. There are four different choices with various combinations of chicken, beef, shrimp, pepperoni, cheese, refried beans, pizza sauce, and some shredded cabbage. We threw that in to make them think it's healthy.

The chicken is fried in the worst fats and is sure to cause heart attacks in at least 50 percent of the consumers. And more good news! The government has ruled that the oil used can be identified on the packaging as tropical oil so unsophisticated consumers will think they're getting something fried in the so-called "good" fat. It actually clogs the arteries twice as fast as the trans fats everybody's talking about these days.

Now for dessert! It's the pièce de résistance. My crafty chefs have created a new mile-high pie that serves two. This delicacy is a sugar addict's dream. It's like having German chocolate cake, a hot fudge sundae, and pecan pie all rolled into one. We call it "Dream Delight." But "Diagnosis Death" is a more apt description. It has corn syrup, high fructose corn syrup, dextrose, sucrose, and we've added a smidgeon of fruit juice for the health fanatics. This product is guaranteed to cause a diabetic to lose a limb or two if we're lucky.

General Drug 'Em Up: We're winning on the healthcare front hands down. A cute pharmaceutical sales rep for one of the major drug companies has just informed hospital administrators in fourteen major cities that a new drug is coming out to help folks who have lactose intolerance. It was tested on laboratory rats and 65 percent of them died! Isn't that wonderful?

The drug does work for a brief period. But it comes with some of the best side effects you could imagine — blindness, sleeplessness, water retention, weight gain, and skin rashes. Twenty percent of the lab rats that lived showed these side effects. Even so, the feds gave the product a green light because the drug company spread around a lot of money and convinced them the dosage consumed by the lab rats was much higher than what humans would ingest.

All of this sounds a bit too dramatic, doesn't it? But when you couple our failure to take full charge of our health with Satan's keen interest in killing us off, the scenarios above begin to sound more plausible. They are by no means meant to glorify the enemy but to expose his plot and raise awareness about the spiritual side of today's "healthcare crisis." All we hear about is the natural side. It is time to dig deeper into this issue so members of the body of Christ can reverse this situation.

Almost everywhere you turn people are either talking about healthcare, or dealing with their own sicknesses or that of ailing family members. We often characterize it as the fight between a person and a disease (she's battling cancer, he's fighting heart disease, etc.). But when you consider efforts in the kingdom of darkness to take advantage of people's dietary weaknesses, you begin to see a broader, more sinister plot.

Just look around. Look at your family and friends. Look at yourself. Look at people in your neighborhood, on your job. Look at the general public. Think about news reports on the sharply rising incidents of juvenile diabetes, the "obesity dilemma," and the "battle against breast cancer," to name a few. The state of "un-health" in America — the richest country in the world — is front-page news.

Now look at the church. Look at people in the congregation on any Sunday morning. Obesity is running as rampant in the sanctuary as it is in the greater society. Better yet, review the prayer requests. Listen to those in the prayer lines for healing. Many believers have been diagnosed with cancer, heart disease, hypertension, diabetes, arthritis, and other killer diseases. You might hear, "Pray for Sister so and so. She's in the hospital with complications from diabetes." Or "Sign this card for Brother so and so. He had quadruple bypass surgery last week."

All of this goes on between the amens and the rush to get out of church and beat the crowds to the nearest buffet. At that time, this shell in which we walk around, this temple of the Holy Spirit (1 Corinthians 6:19), becomes a garbage can for every unhealthy food the world has to offer. Our taste buds are momentarily happy but our cells and organs are crying, "I'm hungry!" In this culture, presenting our bodies as "living sacrifice(s)" (Romans 12:1) is a nice Scripture to quote when we're being super spiritual but is not something we live by on a practical level when we sit down to eat.

In fact, *diet* and *exercise* seem to be dirty words to the corporate body of Christ. This subject is the white elephant in the room that no one wants to talk about. How much teaching do you hear from our pulpits about it? If it is taught by the few brave pastors who dare to go there, how often are churchgoers heeding the message? Not very much if the physical evidence is any indication. By and large, it seems this subject is off-limits at sermon time. But if a pastor looked over his congregation one Sunday and saw half the members were high on cocaine or drunk on alcohol, there is no way he would remain silent about it. Clergy members are good about calling on the Almighty to heal people but rarely urge the saints to stop undermining healing with unhealthy lifestyles.

One night I (Christine) was talking to a friend who had recently been born again and he said something that startled me. This man is very reserved and shy. He is extremely sensitive to other people's feelings. He called to ask if I was watching Christian television. I said, "Yes, I have it on but the sound is muted." He went on to say the teaching was extremely good. I glanced at the television and saw it was a women's conference with thousands of women in the audience. My friend commented that the teacher was giving a powerfully anointed message that had to be impacting the women's spiritual lives. He then asked me, "But why doesn't (the preacher) say something about their bodies? There are a lot of big women in that audience. Just watch when the camera pans the crowd."

I was kind of embarrassed and did not know quite what to say. My first instinct was to defend the women and say their sizes did not matter as long as they were worshiping the Lord. But religious platitudes failed me. This was not an issue of size in terms of what looks good or what meets the world's definition of beauty. It was glaring evidence of open doors to sickness, disease, and heartache. All I could say when I looked at the TV screen was, "You're right."

This insight into the wellness problem facing the church came from a new believer. I thought of the oft-quoted expression from Psalm 8:2 "out of the mouth of babes." I had been in the church all my life but had not realized that many Christians do not pay attention to their health *before* they get sick. It took a new believer, uninitiated in church culture, to point this out to me. The magnitude of this struggle hit home at that moment and has been ever before me since that time.

What do the unsaved think when they see believers battling nutrition related diseases or conditions? Do they wonder about our credibility as we proclaim ourselves as God's "victorious" ambassadors on earth? Do they question our discipline and commitment to the faith we declare? Does the state of our "un-health" distract them from the gospel message? Yes, "faith comes by hearing, and hearing by the word of God" (Romans 10:17). But it surely does not hurt if God's witnesses show forth the fruit of faith, including good health. Yet, in our time, the saints and the non-saints continue to struggle with weight problems and related sicknesses.

The London-based International Obesity Task Force reported in 2003 that two-thirds of American adults are considered overweight. And approximately 300 million people around the world are obese (defined as at least 20 percent greater than a healthy weight) and 750 million more are overweight. This includes 22 million children who are less than five years old. One out of eight school-aged children is obese and one in four is overweight. Obesity among kids has doubled since 1968. In fact, a March 2004 health report written by Duke University researchers and commissioned by the New York based Foundation for Child Development says obesity is the single most widespread health problem facing U.S. children, outpacing accidents and illegal drugs. Obesity is the second leading cause of preventable death in the United States after tobacco.

According to the Center for Disease Control (CDC), diabetes has increased 700 percent since 1959. Each year, 800,000 people are diagnosed with the disease in the United States. In 2005, it was estimated that 20.8 million Americans suffered from diabetes, which is the seventh leading cause of death in the U.S. Of that number, about 6.2 million don't even know they have it. Twenty-one percent (about 40 million) of the U.S. population ages 40-74 is pre-diabetic. Seventy percent of people with diabetes have high blood pressure. Seventy-five percent of diabetics die from heart disease or stroke. The World Health Organization calls diabetes "the fastest growing disease on planet earth."

The National Heart, Lung and Blood Institute estimates that 65 million Americans have high blood pressure and nearly 20 million do not even know they have this condition. Officials with the American Heart Association report that 70 million Americans have cardiovascular disease – the leading cause of U.S. deaths. Every thirty-three seconds, someone dies of heart disease.

Then there is the big "C" – also known as cancer. The World Health Organization says it is the leading cause of death worldwide causing 7.6 million (or 13%) of all deaths around the globe in 2005. The Center for Disease Control (CDC) reported 564,830 people in the U.S. died of cancer in 2006 and has estimated 1.4 million new cases will be reported in America in 2007. The National Cancer Institute and the CDC forecast that within the next decade, cancer is likely to replace heart disease as the biggest killer of those under 75. These agencies report cancer as the leading cause of death among children, thirty-somethings and all ages in between.

An estimated 46 million adults in the U.S. have been diagnosed with some form of arthritis, rheumatoid arthritis, gout, lupus or fibromyalgia according to 2006 Arthritis Foundation data. Over 40% of them or nearly 19 million are limited in their activities because of these conditions. The CDC says "arthritis is the leading cause of disability in the United States." By 2030, the number of doctor-diagnosed arthritis cases is expected to reach 64.9 million.

Our bodies are breaking down in increasingly large numbers! Yet the prevailing solution is to pop a pill or have surgery. Meanwhile, healthcare costs are spiraling. Do you doubt that this is a battle that desperately needs to be won? And it needs to be won at its root — not just cosmetically on the surface, but deep down in the pit of spiritual darkness where it starts.

God desires that we prosper and be in health. Satan wants the opposite. Does this mean there is a devil behind every doughnut? A better question might be, "Does frequently eating doughnuts line up with God's plan that we prosper and be in health or Satan's plan to destroy us?" An honest answer to this question makes the scope of this conflict abundantly clear.

While the body of Christ ignores this very important issue, many people who follow other spiritual disciplines seem to be much better informed about how to stay physically healthy. "ABC News" journalist Diane Sawyer even did a special report on this subject. Her story listed the religions with the slimmest people as Judaism, Islam, Hindu, and Buddhism, and the heaviest religious groups as Baptists, Methodists, Protestants, and Catholics. Overall, Sawyer reported, "Religious Americans are more likely to be overweight than most (other) Americans."

In the August 2006 issue of *Spirituality & Health*, author Alison Buckholtz writes the following in an article entitled "How You Can Help Pastor Your Pastor":

> Studies of Christian clergy's health show that the percentage of clergy who are overweight and therefore at risk for serious disease is higher than that of the U.S. population. One study conducted by the Evangelical Lutheran Church in America and the Mayo Clinic found high percentages of clergy and seminarians at risk due to poor nutrition (72 percent); overweight (64 percent); and hypertension (60 percent). Mirroring these findings, a national survey of more than 2,500 religious leaders conducted in 2004 by Pulpit & Pew, a research project on pastoral leadership based in Duke Divinity School, found that 76 percent of Christian clergy were either overweight or obese, compared with 61 percent of the general population.

This magazine's contents — according to its mission statement — are drawn from "the wisdom of many traditions and cultures with an emphasis on sharing spiritual practices." Some editions include articles on astrology and other non-Christian spiritual practices as well as advertisements for businesses that offer neurofeedback healing, Zen clocks, intuitive healing, yoga classes, Buddhist retreats, Reiki (a "spiritual healing art"), "spiritual deepening programs," and a variety of other alternative or non-traditional health practices including new age disciplines.

It should be troublesome to Christians that non-Christians do a better job of taking care of their physical health than members of the body of Christ. We should be at the forefront of this movement and should have the results to back it up, just like Jesus did. Author Joyce Rogers puts it this way in her book, *The Bible's Seven Secrets To Healthy Eating*, "Most Christians know far less about good nutrition than some members of false religions."

When I (Christine) took an Asian tour in 2004, I encountered many wonderful people of mostly non-Christian faiths. Most of them — young and old — were thin and fit. The majority of them ride bikes and can squat on the ground for long periods of time in a position few Westerners past puberty could manage. But their bathrooms tell the real story of our different levels of fitness. The comments I had heard about their "holes in the ground" were not exaggerated. The toilets are clearly designed for the fit and nimble. There were no handrails or anything to help you squat or get up! I often heard people in my tour group ask, "Do they have any Western-style bathrooms in this place?"

On many occasions, the answer was no, as it was at one rest stop outside of Beijing. A lady traveling with us who was very obese went to the restroom. On my way in, I met her on the way out. She had a very distressed look on her face. I asked, "What's wrong?" She replied sadly, "They don't have any Western bathroom stalls in this place." She was dressed in slacks, which would have made it even harder for her to use the bathroom. It was a very awkward moment. I did not know how to help her use the bathroom. It would have taken at least two people to assist her. I said, "Maybe we'll stop again before we get to the hotel" and quickly rushed past her into the bathroom. When I came out, I saw her in the convenience store buying ice cream.

In these predominantly Muslim and Buddhist nations I visited, they bragged about their vegetarian diets and gave tours of their religious temples. I noticed the images of livestock on the roofs of these buildings and could not help but think how meat from the animals they hold sacred end up on our plates two or three times a day in America. It was a very sobering moment. In one country, I was told the government actually endorses the mostly vegetable and grain-based diets eaten by the vast majority of citizens.

Now don't close the book and go screaming into the night! I am not telling anyone to become a vegetarian. I am simply pointing out some cultural and spiritual differences and the irony of it all. Some Christians — who profess allegiance to the Great Physician — are not as physically healthy as some non-Christians. And those of us who live in Western countries are the most challenged in this area. One can't help but wonder what Jesus thinks about all this.

I was reminded a number of times during that trip that Americans are not as healthy as Asians. The Chinese did not hesitate to point this out. A Chinese tour guide who was giving us some information about popular attractions in Beijing said, "Tiananmen Square is the largest public square in the world — capable of holding one million people." She then paused and barely suppressing a giggle said, "That's one million Chinese but only 500,000 Americans." An employee at our hotel told us, "Cabs in Beijing are very small. Some of you may want to have the hotel concierge order a number twenty-seven cab for you. That's a larger car and you will be able to fit. Otherwise, you will not be able to fit in the regular taxis."

What are the Chinese doing differently? For one thing, their diet is very low in fat, yet high in plant-based foods, such as fruits, vegetables, and soy products. Could Americans learn a dietary lesson from the Chinese? You bet. The Chinese certainly think so and they have the statistics to back it up.

T. Colin Campbell, Ph.D., and Christine Cox write in their book *The China Project* that only four in every 100,000 males under age sixty-five in China die of heart disease each year, while sixty-seven out of 100,000 die in the United States. This book summarizes the results of comprehensive studies done in China in 1983 and 1989 to determine whether varying diets in different parts of China would correlate to death rates from certain diseases. The diets of 10,200 Chinese and Taiwanese adults and their families were assessed. The findings confirm the link between diet and disease.

- The highest cholesterol levels in rural China were near the lowest levels found in the United States.
- Even at these low cholesterol levels, those at the higher end of the Chinese range had significantly more cancer and heart disease than those at the lower end.
- A high blood level of cholesterol was consistently associated with many cancers — including leukemia, liver, colon, rectum, lung, and brain.
- The incidence of death from heart disease is seventeen times higher for American men than Chinese.
- The Chinese eat almost no dairy products and low levels of calcium-rich foods, yet get less osteoporosis than we do in the West.

- The Chinese eat almost three hundred more calories than we do per day yet far fewer Chinese are obese.
- In China, the more fiber eaten, the lower the rate of bowel cancer.
- Men in China had the lowest advanced prostate cancer rates in the world — one in every 100,000 men — while Chinese-American men living in San Francisco had a rate nineteen times as high.
- The highest rates of breast cancer occur in the countries where people eat the most meat.

These are impressive statistics. But on the spiritual side, people in some Eastern cultures follow healthcare practices that are rooted in philosophies contrary to Christian beliefs. Therapies associated with Eastern religions include: hypnosis, Reiki, Tai Chi, Therapeutic Touch, so-called "energy medicines," Transcendental Meditation, some massage therapies, and color therapy to name a few. Although nicely packaged and perhaps physically beneficial on some level, these alternative therapies could open those who use them to new age teachings such as religious ceremonies to solicit help with a health problem from pagan gods.

Dónal O'Mathúna, Ph.D., and Walt Larimore, M.D., warn in *Alternative Medicine, The Christian Handbook*:

> Some alternative therapies refer to the spirit in ways that are alien to Christianity. Unless you understand the roots of a particular therapy, you may find yourself involved in a practice with a theology dangerously different from what Jesus taught or what He would have us follow.

O'Mathúna and Larimore caution that certain practitioners of alternative medicine may follow these beliefs and try to convert their patients to these philosophies. Their book gives an overview of several holistic medicine therapies, including their religious perspectives.

Once again we can see this struggle is both physical *and* spiritual. Yet another irony! Christians have solid spiritual food but many of us have shaky diets. Some non-believers have good diets and fitness regimens but shaky spiritual beliefs! It just goes to show you, Satan hates everybody and will mess up your life with whatever brand of poison you'll allow!

Perhaps some Christians do not see the seriousness of our healthcare situation because they believe focusing on it too much could lead to glorifying the flesh. They might rely on John 6:63 where Jesus, speaking to the disciples, said, "It is the Spirit who gives life; the flesh profits nothing." It is true. The flesh profits nothing in that no work of the flesh can save you from your sins. But this is not a license to let the flesh fall into disrepair. Although it is not the source of life, the flesh is the house where the human spirit and soul — the real person — resides while we live on the earth. So the body has a significant role to play in spiritual matters. The Son of God had to use one to get his work done on earth, and so do we.

The Bible also says, "The life of the flesh is in the blood" (Leviticus 17:11). There are two key messages in this passage: 1) spiritual life is in the blood of Jesus, for he washes away our sins and 2) natural life is in the blood flowing through our veins. It washes away toxins or poisons that can cause sickness and disease and carries nutrients throughout our body. That's why one of the first things doctors do at a physical is draw blood so they can have it analyzed to rule out various health conditions. That's why people die when the heart stops and blood is no longer pumped to vital organs. That's why it is said, "You are what you eat." What you eat determines your blood condition, which determines your organ condition, which determines how you live and — barring accidents or intentional violence — how you die.

Satan uses deception to try to keep people away from both of these blood benefits. He blinds them to the sin cleansing power of Jesus' blood. And he blinds them to the danger of a corrupt food supply system or holds them in such bondage to it that they feel they cannot fight the temptation to eat killer foods. The bottom line is this: Satan is out for blood. But death due to diet will not happen if believers are geared for combat as the apostle Paul instructed. After identifying Satan as our enemy in Ephesians 6:11-12, he went on to write:

> ***Therefore take up the whole armor of God, that you may be able to withstand in the evil day, and having done all, to stand. Stand therefore, having girded your waist with truth, having put on the breastplate of righteousness, and having shod your feet with the preparation of the gospel of peace; above all, taking the shield of faith with which you will be able to quench all the fiery darts of the wicked one. And take the helmet of salvation, and the sword of the Spirit, which is***

the word of God; praying always with all prayer and supplication in the Spirit, being watchful to this end with all perseverance and supplication for all the saints.
~ Ephesians 6:13-18

Truth, faith, the Word of God, and prayer are essential weapons in the fight to live victoriously — including the struggle for physical wellness. Pursuing truth will help us see the danger in some products marketed by a food industry bent on making money from the sale of goods that are harmful to people's health. The word of God hidden in the heart will crush cravings for nutritionally bankrupt food. And prayer keeps us in relationship with the giver of life and focused on what he called us to do. Since our calling is to dominate the earth in all areas of life, what better place to start than in the area of health and nutrition?

It is time for members of the body of Christ to stop perishing on the health battlefield simply because we have not grasped the spiritual scope of this struggle and therefore are not tackling it like spiritual warriors. Now is the time to stop relying on the world's weapons in this fight. Satan likes to see us use them and fail so he can try to make a mockery of God's covenant people. But it shall not be so! We must set ourselves apart in the healthcare war and shine forth as the overcomers we are destined to be thanks to the Blood of the Lamb.

Every day when we eat right and exercise regularly, we rule the roost. When we do not, we give the forces of darkness an opportunity to take charge of our health. Frankly, it is simply unacceptable for God's people to allow a defeated devil to manipulate us into routinely presenting our bodies as receptacles for toxic foods, prescription drugs, and fresh meat for the surgeon's scalpel. Yet here we are, members of the only organization called to warfare that is passive about getting prepared. But you cannot get prepared if you don't know what is at stake, don't know your enemy, and don't know your enemy's tactics. Satan has a long history of tricking us into self-destruction. The next chapter deals with how it all got started — ironically enough — with food.

Chapter Summary

1. Many members of the body of Christ are struggling in the area of diet and wellness just like thousands of unbelievers.
2. Satan goes to great extremes to get people to destroy themselves with food, as is reflected by the rise in diet-related diseases and conditions.
3. Studies indicate many Western Christians tend to be more overweight and/or unhealthy than members of other religions.
4. Some health practices associated with Eastern religions get good physical results but can open the door to non-Christian belief systems.
5. The children of God must:
   a. Recognize the battle for health is physical, mental and spiritual.
   b. Get spiritually strengthened to win it.
   c. Continuously set a better health example for the rest of the world.

Chapter Three

Abandoned Authority

You have made him to have dominion over the works of Your hands; You have put all things under his feet.
~ Psalm 8:6

Lord I thank you for this food I am about to receive for the nourishment of my body for Christ's sake. Amen.

Anyone who has been around church folk at mealtime has probably heard this prayer. It meets all the religious requirements. The Lord is acknowledged. "Thanks" is given. And the prayer is closed with the proper "Amen". Meanwhile, mouths water. Eyes sparkle at the sight of the food all laid out. Noses inhale the aroma of what is expected to be a pleasurable experience. And hands are eager to dig in. When the flesh is fully engaged like this, "blessing the food" is sometimes a jumble of quickly spoken words — a routinely pious exercise leading up to the main event. This way the person saying grace won't annoy people who don't like long-winded petitions to God standing between them and their favorite dishes.

In any event, the words of this prayer definitely make the connection between diet and destiny, such as "Nourishment ... for Christ's sake." To "nourish" according to *Webster's Dictionary* means to "nurture, rear, maintain, support, feed, furnish, or sustain nutriment." Nurture means "to further the development of." Nutriment means "something that nourishes or promotes growth and repairs the natural wastage of organic life." Wastage means "loss, decrease, or destruction of something (as by use, decay, erosion, or leakage) especially wasteful or avoidable loss of something valuable."

So to tell God at mealtime you are nourishing yourself "for Christ's sake" makes what you eat very serious business. Furthermore, the phrase, "This food that I am about to receive for the nourishment of my body ..." is a statement that makes nutrition a distinctly personal responsibility. If you make sure your meals are truly nourishing, then hopefully you will be on the planet long enough and have enough energy to make a contribution to the work for which Christ gave his life. If not, you have not been a good steward over your flesh and may very well have opened the door to a preventable sickness or disease.

This is *how* the body of Christ gets beaten in the health and nutrition war day after day. But the bigger question is *why* do we lose this fight so often? Believers who have accepted Jesus Christ as Lord and Savior have the right and power to exercise control over every challenge in life — including anything that can undermine good health. Jesus gave us this power.

> *For you are all sons of God through faith in Christ Jesus.*
> *~ Galatians 3:26*

> *Behold, I give you the authority to trample on serpents and scorpions, and over all the power of the enemy, and nothing shall by any means hurt you. ~ Luke 10:19*

Therefore, Christians who cannot control appetites of any kind have an authority problem. They either do not know they have power to influence or command thought or behavior, or they know it but do not know how to exercise these rights. So what happens when believers are faced with a dietary temptation that can potentially destroy good health? It depends on what they think.

If people make no connection between what they routinely eat and long-term health, then they will not exercise any authority over urges to eat nutritionally bankrupt food. This is unfortunate because you cannot fight an enemy you do not see or overcome one you ignore. Even worse, some Christians believe getting sick with diseases like cancer, diabetes, and hypertension as they age is just part of the normal life cycle.

There are other believers who are more proactive. They try to stay fit by following the latest and greatest new diet they saw on TV or read about in a magazine. They might hold out for a couple of months, if that long, before they start cheating. Eventually, they feel bad about going off their diet, throw up their hands, and wait for the next weight loss program promoted by some Hollywood celebrity or new age fitness guru. Round and round we go. We continuously look to the world for answers instead of our Maker. This is that nasty little habit handed down to us by Adam and Eve.

Before the fall, they were built to live forever in a perfect setting. They were in charge of everything.

> *Then God blessed them, and God said to them, "Be fruitful and multiply; fill the earth and subdue it; have dominion over the fish of the sea, over the birds of the air, and over every living thing that moves on the earth." ~ Genesis 1:28*

Death was only mentioned in the context of sin. And temptation was tied to the produce of one tree. But every other fruit and vegetable was available to them for food.

> *And God said, "See, I have given you every herb that yields seed which is on the face of all the earth, and every tree whose fruit yields seed to you it shall be for food."*
> *~ Genesis 1:29*

> *And out of the ground the Lord God made every tree grow that is pleasant to the sight and good for food. The tree of life was also in the midst of the garden, and the tree of the knowledge of good and evil. ~ Genesis 2:9*

> *And the Lord commanded the man, saying, "Of every tree of the garden you may freely eat; but of the tree of the knowledge of good and evil you shall not eat, for in the day that you eat of it you shall surely die." ~ Genesis 2:16-17*

Satan, disguised as a serpent, directed Eve's attention to the forbidden fruit just as television and other advertisements today direct our attention to foods we should not eat. He asked, "Has God indeed said, 'You shall not eat of every tree of the garden?'" (Genesis 3:1). Before that moment, there is no indication in Scripture that Eve had desired the tree's food. Once her attention was drawn to it, she did not rebuke the idea or thought but said, "We may eat the fruit of the trees of the garden; but of the fruit of the tree which is in the midst of the garden, God has said, 'You shall not eat it, nor shall you touch it, lest you die.'" (Genesis 3:2-3)

Sitting here comfortably in the church age, we have the ability to meditate on Eve's situation and learn from her mistakes. First of all, she almost had the right idea. She spoke some of God's Word but added the part about "nor shall you touch it." In addition, her response focused too much on a negative fact — the forbidden tree — and not God's whole truth, which included the tree of life. Her reply was rather passive and certainly not the kind of response you would expect from a woman who shared control of the whole earth with her husband. There was not much conviction in it and absolutely no power at all. What if she had said the following?

> I rebuke thee, O serpent, and bind your efforts to direct my attention to a tree God has forbidden for food. I shall not eat of it and I shall not die. God has given me the tree of life from which to eat. It is more than enough. I rule and reign in this garden with my husband, Adam, and you have no power or rights here to control me or anything in this place. Be off with you, liar and accuser of the brethren.

If Eve had exercised her God-given rights and sent the serpent packing, the subject of this book would be a non-issue and we would all probably be sitting around in paradise eating untainted food without having to work hard for it. We would no doubt be communing with the Almighty in the cool of the garden and patting lions on the head without fear. But at that crossroad between obedience and desire, Eve chose her flesh over her future. Here's what led to that fatal decision.

After the enemy planted the idea in Eve's head that the fruit on the wrong tree would be good for her, she developed a desire for it. You will notice it was "fruit" — something sweet — and not broccoli that tempted Eve. She then ate and gave some to Adam (Genesis 3:6). They did not eat the forbidden fruit because they had no other choices. God had more than amply provided for their dietary needs. They ate it because they saw it and it *looked* good. They did not exercise their God-given authority and quench their desire. Now, let's look at what we all lost over a snack.

Eating the fruit of one tree cost them everything. They lost their spiritual oneness with God. They lost their legacy of dominion over the earth. They lost their perfect habitat and brought a curse on all creation. They lost immortality. Ultimately it was an extremely expensive meal. Using a modern day expression, we might say these were some seriously "empty calories"!

So here we have it. Mankind's very first sin on earth was related to food — something that sits on the tongue for a few seconds, passes through the intestines, and is virtually forgotten until its remnants come out the other end as waste. For this the earth was sent into a tailspin. Everything that has happened here since that time is the result of that one ill-fated meal. The choice was to fight or fall, and Adam and Eve chose to fall.

What did they gain? Nothing. Presumably their eyes and taste buds were briefly satisfied, but for what? A quick thrill in exchange for a lifetime of despair and millennia of misery for their offspring! Their once immortal bodies became mortal — susceptible to deterioration, disease, and death. They experienced shame. "Then the eyes of both of them were opened, and they knew that they were naked; and they sewed fig leaves together and made themselves coverings" (Genesis 3:7).

Once they became flesh conscious, they covered their physique — including the parts that identified them as male and female. Having lost their authority they became confused about their identities and their place in the world. Before the fall, clothes were not an issue because they were not programmed to focus on their physical appearance. But after the fall, their natural senses of sight, touch, smell, hearing, and taste dominated. They had lost the connection with God's revelation power.

Fear also came upon Adam and Eve. When God came looking for them, Adam said, "I heard Your voice in the garden and I was afraid because I was naked; and I hid myself" (Genesis 3:10). Then came strife and an unrepentant spirit, for Adam said, "The woman whom You gave to be with me, she gave me of the tree, and I ate" (Genesis 3:12). Adam was basically saying it was someone else's fault and if you don't buy that excuse, God, then it is your fault for putting me in this marriage with this woman. There is no indication Adam or Eve showed any remorse for disobeying God.

And then came the curses. Adam, Eve, and the serpent each received one. All three curses involved some aspect of eating or appetites.

The serpent: "And you shall eat dust all the days of your life" (Genesis 3:14). This means the serpent would crawl on its belly forever. It's believed the serpent had legs before this curse was invoked.

The woman: "Your desire shall be for your husband. And he shall rule over you" (Genesis 3:16). I (Christine) have heard the latter part of this passage interpreted by one pastor to mean the woman would compete with her husband for his place of headship or authority.

The man: "Cursed is the ground for your sake; In toil you shall eat of it all the days of your life. Both thorns and thistles it shall bring forth for you, and you shall eat the herb of the field. In the sweat of your face you shall eat bread till you return to the ground" (Genesis 3:17-19).

From that time on, man has had to work hard to help meet his dietary needs — from planting and harvesting crops, to raising livestock, to working twelve-hour days on a modern day job. But the ultimate curse was death — spiritual and physical. This meal spiritually separated Adam and Eve from God and eventually led to physical death. This is our first nutrition lesson. The wrong food can kill you.

Fast forward several generations and we can see how their legacy of no appetite control continued to cause damage in the lives of succeeding generations. Esau, the grandson of the Hebrew patriarch Abraham, also fell prey to a dietary temptation. And just like Adam and Eve, he forfeited his future for some food.

> *Jacob was boiling pottage (lentil stew) one day, when Esau came from the field and was faint [with hunger]. And Esau said to Jacob, "I beg of you, let me have some of that red lentil stew to eat, for I am faint and famished." ... Jacob answered, "Then sell me today your birthright (the rights of a firstborn)." Esau said, "See here, I am at the point of death; what good can this birthright do me?" Jacob said, "Swear to me today [that you are selling it to me]"; and he swore to [Jacob] and sold him his birthright. Then Jacob gave Esau bread and stew of lentils, and he ate and drank and rose up and went his way. Thus Esau scorned his birthright as beneath his notice. ~ Genesis 25:29-34 (AMP)*

A birthright represented authority and headship in a family. Recipients received a double portion from their fathers as an inheritance. When Esau gave up his birthright he abandoned his position of authority and Jacob took it.

Several centuries later, Satan — with no new tricks up his sleeve — tried tempting Jesus with food. After a forty-day fast in the wilderness, Jesus was hungry.

> *Now when the tempter came to Him, he said, "If You are the Son of God, command that these stones become bread." But he answered and said, "It is written, 'Man shall not live by*

bread alone, but by every word that proceeds from the mouth of God." ~ Matthew 4:3-4

Finally, a new precedent was set. Jesus exemplified the right way to deal with temptation including food temptations. He used his authority and held Satan in check by quoting the Word of God as set forth in Deuteronomy 8:3. The chaos that came about after Adam and Eve failed to control their appetites was now on the way to being reversed. Jesus put it this way:

The Spirit of the Lord is upon Me, Because He has anointed Me to preach the gospel to the poor; He has sent Me to heal the brokenhearted, to proclaim liberty to the captives and recovery of sight to the blind, to set at liberty those who are oppressed; to proclaim the acceptable year of the Lord.
~ Luke 4:18-19

The King of Kings bought back the authority the first man and woman so frivolously gave away in the Garden. He did this when he laid down his life on the cross at Calvary and rose from the dead on the third day morning. Before he ascended to heaven to sit at the right hand of God the Father, Jesus declared, "All authority has been given to Me in heaven and on earth" (Matthew 28:18). He destroyed "the works of the devil" (1 John 3:8) and reinstated here on earth the rights of citizens of the kingdom of God.

As joint heirs with Christ (Romans 8:17), those reborn from above, according to John 3:16, now have the right to reign as God's stewards in this divine government. This includes operating God's way by speaking his Word and addressing trouble with truth. Christians armed in this manner can stand against satanic plots designed to lure them into acts of disobedience and destruction — even at the dinner table.

Once we recognize this authority and begin to use it, we can change our lives in the natural realm — including our dietary habits. But knowing you have this right and exercising it are two different things. If the police chief in your town deputized you, gave you a gun and badge, and authorized you to arrest criminals, it would do you no good if you came upon a car thief and just stood by and watched him or her take your car.

It's the same with our God-given authority. We must use it to keep our appetites in check, including the same temptations that trapped Adam and Eve. Otherwise, we end up relying on our flesh instead of relying on our spirit. We end up chasing after every new health fad the world tries to sell us — instead of asking God exactly what meal plan he wants us to follow. Author John Bevere puts it this way in his book *Breaking Intimidation*: "If you don't walk in your God-given authority, someone will take if from you and use it against you." I (Christine) was reminded of this teaching in late 2003 when Annie, one of my mother's good friends, died at the age of seventy.

I had known Annie most of my life. She was well known and well liked in our small, rural community. She was a pleasant, jovial, church-going woman. As long as I had known Annie she had always been obese. About a year before her death, she was diagnosed with uterine cancer. The doctors performed surgery and gave her radiation treatment. A few months before her death, Annie began to feel very sick again. My mom told me, "She was always complaining about feeling a lot of tightness in her chest. She would be hungry but could not eat without feeling sick. Whenever she ate something greasy — like fried chicken — she could not keep it down."

Annie was encouraged to go back to the doctor but she said she did not have the money. When offered money, Annie still refused to go. Instead, she took a lot of over-the-counter medication, trying to relieve her symptoms. One night, Annie got terribly sick and was rushed to the hospital. Shortly after she was admitted, the doctor announced Annie had stomach cancer. A short time later, he advised the family she was brain dead. Soon thereafter, he reported she had had a heart attack. And then she died.

My mother was terribly distraught. She blamed the ER doctors, saying, "She should have had her family doctor there. Those ER doctors aren't any good." She then blamed the red tape of the Medicaid system that deemed Annie ineligible — supposedly because she "owned a lot of land." I could not help but wonder at what point in Annie's seventy years had her body started going downhill in that direction. Did anyone ever tell her that as a God-fearing, born-again, Bible believing, church-going Christian she had the authority and power to take charge of this situation as part of her birthright?

I (Christine) don't know the answer to these questions, but I do know adopting a healthy lifestyle is doable God's way. Again, it starts with exercising the authority he gave us for our edification and not for destruction. (2 Corinthians 10:8). *Edification* means to build or establish; to instruct and improve especially in moral and religious knowledge; to enlighten. Although we have the right to choose what we eat, we are nevertheless responsible for making sure we use this power of choice to build ourselves up and not destroy ourselves.

What would Jesus say about the bodies in the body of Christ today? Maybe he would say something like this:

My children, I died a brutal death for you so you would not have to. Yet you still allow the evils of a fallen planet to rule over your flesh and destroy it cell by cell. Remember, children, I redeemed you from all of this. I have reversed Adam's curse. Now you just have to walk in the authority gained by my sacrifice. Why are you not accepting my entire gift? Why is your soul not prospering so that your body can, too? Why are you letting your divine destiny be interrupted with conditions as bad or worse than those I walked from village to village to heal? Do you not know the scope of your inheritance? Don't you know it was the image of you living victoriously that I saw when I was on that cross? That is why I did not come down, even when the soldiers taunted me. Love and my vision for your future is what kept me on that tree. I endured the pain so that you could be free. Take up the gift. Rule and reign as you are ordained to do. Reclaim your health now and carry out my great commission whole and unhindered! God's kingdom needs willing hearts and able bodies.

Begin today exercising all of your spiritual authority and power to nourish and preserve your temple. Do it for Christ's sake.

Chapter Summary

1. The whole world fell under a curse when Adam and Eve did not resist a snack recommended by Satan.
2. Jesus' sacrifice on the cross reversed the curse of sin and got back for us the authority we need to overcome life's challenges including those related to physical health.
3. Christians must begin to use this authority to fight sickness and disease and stay healthy for the sake of God's kingdom work.

Chapter Four

Does It Really Run in the Family?

*Everything a man naturally inherits from his parents belongs
to the flesh.* ~ Watchman Nee, The Spiritual Man

I (Christine) was angrier than the victim. As unbelievable as it was, she was not even upset about the ugly scar left on her stomach after her husband sliced her mid-section from one side to the other and beat her until she was black and blue. Instead, she was mad at me for "locking up her man." She stuck to her story, too. "I cut myself while preparing a chicken for dinner," she said.

I saw many women like her during the time I worked as an assistant district attorney. After a while, most of the justice system's problems (bad judges, lying defendants, unjust verdicts, etc.) rolled off my back. But I never forgot the crime victim's wounds. Cuts, bruises, gunshot injuries, cigarette burns on babies — these I never forgot. During closing arguments, I reminded jurors of the pain my victim suffered and demanded a conviction and punishment for the defendant that fit the crime.

That is exactly how I felt when I saw my Aunt Sallie a few years ago. I wanted to lock up someone! But there are no jail cells for diseases. Diabetes had attacked her in mid-life. By the time I saw her that spring day at her home in Phoenix, the disease had taken one of her eyes, one of her big toes, and both kidneys. She was going for dialysis three times a week. I had not seen her in about ten years. When I looked at her, I was so startled I literally gasped. I put my hand over my mouth and thought, *My goodness, she looks like she's been mugged!*

Aunt Sallie was one of those relatives you were always glad to see — even as a kid. She was one of my favorites — happy, quick-witted, and with a sense of humor that always left my sides aching from laughter every time I saw her. Not even the diabetes could take that away. One of the first jokes she cracked when I saw her on that visit was about not being able to wear sandals anymore because she was missing a toe. Aunt Sallie was a good wife and mother who worked hard all of her life.

She was a beautiful person inside and out, humble and down to earth. She never put on any airs and I don't believe she knew how pretty she really was. She had flawless skin, and bright greenish-gray eyes touched with kindness and a hint of mischief. For her to lose one of them to diabetic complications was just incomprehensible to me! But being robbed of one of her best features was just one of many attacks she suffered from this dreaded disease. On Thursday, November 16, 2006, my Aunt Sallie's struggle with her condition ended and she transitioned to her eternal home.

If you don't think staying healthy is like being in a war, a photograph of my Aunt Sallie before and after diabetes will change your mind. This is a woman who did everything the doctors told her to do after she was diagnosed. She lost weight and kept it off — not that she had ever had much of a weight problem. She ate what the doctors told her to eat. One of the last things she said to me during my visit to her home was, "Child, I'm fightin' hard to stay in this world."

Two of her daughters struggle with this same disease. Again, two beautiful and remarkable women, saddled with diabetes. And so it goes, generation after generation, sickness after sickness, death after death, loved one after loved one too often struck down by the same diseases. Why do these things happen? Are they just situations we can't do anything about because we live on an imperfect planet? Are we just frail creatures destined to get sick and then sometimes pass the condition on to our children? In other words, if Grandma and Mama had a disease, will those in the next generation have it, too, no matter how they live? Is there nothing that can be done about it?

Many people don't believe there is anything that can be done about it — including some Christians. They expect to have the same diseases or health problems their ancestors had: diabetes, arthritis, heart disease, hypertension, etc. They are not surprised when it happens just like they are not surprised when they inherit a parent's eye color, mouth, skin tone, walk, or habits. I (Christine) remember how horrified I was one day when my father said, "All of the people in my family have arthritis." I cried out, "It shall not come near me!"

But messages around us suggest it will. The first time you go to a doctor's office for treatment, you are asked to fill out a form with questions about your family medical history. If you reveal that a relative has or had a particular disease, the doctor will consider that information relevant to your diagnosis. He or she might even say something like, "You're at risk for breast cancer because your mom had it" or "You'll need regular check-ups because I see heart disease runs in your family." This just reinforces the idea that if your daddy and his brother had a disease, you'll probably have it, too. But Dr. Aubrey

Milunsky, a medical geneticist at Harvard Medical School, says otherwise in his book *Your Genetic Destiny*. He writes:

> Contrary to popular belief, your genetic destiny is not preordained. True, you are born with a genetic blueprint that dictates the structure and functioning of your body. Notwithstanding this irrevocable fact of nature, you are not a hapless victim, inevitably bound to suffer the inexorable consequences of any flawed genes you may have inherited. Although every aspect of health and all disease is controlled, regulated, modulated, or influenced by your genes, genes are not the last word; there is much more you should know and much you can do to influence the outcome.

Milunsky wrote his book from a secular viewpoint. But it is more optimistic than what you might hear some Christians say about their medical conditions. Their speech about sickness sometimes lines up more with Satan's word than God's Word. Instead of hearing, "I declare in the name of Jesus that my children and their children will not have diabetes even though my husband had it," you might hear them say, "I told my daughter to take my grandson to the doctor because I believe he has diabetes just like his daddy does."

But Dr. Milunsky has a better report. He writes, "All aspects of health and illness are both governed by genes and influenced by environmental factors. The vast majority of disorders that affect mankind are due to interactions between genes and environmental agents such as bacteria and virus, dietary components, and toxins." In other words, we have something to say about how the genes we inherit from our parents interact with natural and supernatural forces.

Let's look at our natural surroundings first. Is your flesh living in hostile or hospitable territory? Is it given the right food, exercise, and rest? Is it getting what it needs to not only overcome genetic flaws, but to thrive? Your health is not simply a matter of just accepting the flesh in which you were born. It also involves how you control the environment in which your body will fight to live. Compare it to a car. The raw materials that go into an automobile might not be perfect, but the vehicle will run a lot better and longer if the owner follows the manufacturer's recommended maintenance schedule for oil changes, tune ups, tire rotations, etc.

Genes are the raw materials for our bodies. God designed them, knit them together in our mother's womb, and gave us maintenance guidelines on how to keep the finished product running while we're living on earth. Genes control the make up of blood and arteries as well as process the chemical elements of food that is eaten. So if we give bad genes bad food to process, we increase the risk of ending up with bad health. Milunsky paints a vivid picture of how genes can impact quality of life:

> Our genes regulate, modify, control, promote, enhance, and otherwise influence every aspect of our body's structure and functioning. Whether you are tall or short, fat or thin, fair- or dark-skinned, have certain facial characteristics, are allergic, or are affected by a genetic disorder is purely a function of your genes. Your genes largely determine your body's characteristics, your various susceptibilities or resistance to all diseases, how you react to medications, and whether you will transmit certain genetic disorders or fall victim to one or more of them. However, even though all aspects of health depend upon your genes, their interaction with the environment is especially important.

Here are some of the major diseases or conditions and controllable environmental factors — including diet — that Milunsky says can aggravate genetic flaws:

Cardiovascular disease — the main cause of death in developed countries.

Environmental factors include: obesity, lack of exercise, high fat diets, and smoking.

High blood pressure (hypertension) — a main risk factor for heart attack, stroke, kidney failure, and other disorders of the blood vessels.

Environmental factors: the presence of diabetes, high blood fats, obesity, excessive alcohol consumption and smoking. Although hypertension commonly occurs within families, studies reveal people suffering from the condition realize the most significant benefit when they stop eating salt and stick to a low-fat diet with lots of fruit and vegetables.

Diabetes — This disease occurs when a person either does not produce enough insulin, a hormone that converts the food we eat into glucose, or they produce enough but, for some reason, the insulin cannot transport the glucose through the blood into cells where it is needed. Studies show it is relatively rare for a single gene to cause diabetes.

The term *diabetes* was first coined by seventeenth century British physician Thomas Willis, who attended the royal family and had a reputation as one of the finest doctors of his time. Author William Dufty describes Willis's work in his book *Sugar Blues*. Dufty notes diabetes became prominent after two hundred years of sugar eating in England. By 1662, consumption of the treat had gone from zero to sixteen million pounds a year.

The United States Department of Agriculture estimates that the average American consumes 20 teaspoons of sugar a day. This might not seem like much to some people but a 12-ounce can of soda contains about 9 teaspoons of sugar. There are conflicting opinions as to whether or not sugar causes or contributes to causing diabetes. But the Harvard School of Public Health issued a press release in 2004 stating that researchers found "women who increased their intake or consumed higher amounts of sugar-sweetened beverages had a greater magnitude of weight gain and a higher risk of developing type 2 diabetes compared to women who consumed fewer sugar-sweetened drinks." In any event, there's no disagreement that certain environmental factors (e.g. obesity, lack of exercise, smoking, high blood fat levels, and consumption of processed foods that raise the blood sugar level too fast) can aggravate diabetes -- a disease that has risen to epidemic proportions in the United States.

Obesity — Genetic constitution might predispose a person to obesity but what they do with that genetic make-up determines whether they are obese or not.

Environmental factors: Culture and diet. Carole Krause, in her book, *How Healthy is Your Family Tree?* says, "If you know the tendency toward being overweight is genetic, you might take diet and nutrition more seriously. As a young person, look at your mother and father and other relatives. Do you see obesity? Then consult a doctor and nutritionist and develop a realistic eating and exercise plan."

Cancer — All cancers involve "genetic machinery," according to Dr. Milunsky, but only about ten percent are truly inherited. And even these can potentially be overcome with proactive health maintenance regimens including "surveillance plans that result in early detection and pre-emptive treatment." Milunsky writes:

> Many people have a pessimistic and fatalistic view about inherited cancer, convinced that they can do nothing about their own risk. Nothing could be further from the truth. Certainly, knowledge of specific cancers in the family should enable those who know their genes to save their lives.

In 2002 the World Health Organization and the United Nation's Food and Agriculture Organization heard from a group of international scientists that some of our favorite foods (French fries, potato chips, and some breakfast cereals) may cause cancer. These foods reportedly contain high levels of a substance called acrylamide, which is known to cause cancer in laboratory rats. Nutritionist Dr. Ted Broer — who is also a Christian — says sixty percent of cancers diagnosed in females and forty percent in males is "related to diet and nutrition."

Environmental factors impacting the risk of all cancers: smoking (which accounts for about thirty percent of deaths due to cancer), dietary habits (especially excess fat intake), and other environmental carcinogens.

Environmental factors for breast cancer: use of oral contraceptives for at least ten years and high alcohol intake (three or more drinks per day).

Environmental factors for colon cancer (only 3 to 5 percent of cases are thought to have a direct genetic link): chronic inflammatory diseases of the bowel and high-fat, low-fiber diets.

Environmental factors for prostate cancer: obesity, red meat and fat consumption, and certain toxins.

Alzheimer's Disease — Only about ten percent of all cases of Alzheimer's are directly inherited/transmitted via a single gene.

Environmental factors: Malnutrition (even mild and transient) during the brain maturation years, growing up in a low socioeconomic area and having multiple siblings, and cigarette smoking.

That's the story from the natural side of life. Now let's look at the supernatural side of this sickness inheritance problem. Adam and Eve released a curse on the earth when they disobeyed God and ate forbidden fruit in the Garden of Eden. A curse is evil or misfortune that comes in response to something said or done. The something "done" in Adam and Eve's case was they ate food God told them not to eat.

They not only brought a curse on themselves and all their descendants (see Romans 5:12) but on the earth as well. Genesis 3:17 reads: "The ground is under a curse because of you" (AMP). Romans 8:20 describes the earth as being "subjected to frailty" and "condemned to frustration" (AMP). In other words, the earth changed from a paradise to a hazard zone. In some respects, it became a toxic and hostile environment. We face danger from tornadoes, hurricanes, earthquakes, blizzards, droughts, floods, certain animal and plant life, toxins, viruses, bacteria, etc. Some of these are the conditions Dr. Milunsky calls "environmental factors." From the supernatural perspective, they are consequences of the Adamic curse.

With these curse conditions running loose on earth, there is potential for bad things to happen to good and not so good people. Why? Because they either do something to invite a bad situation into their lives or they are faced with a bad situation and do nothing on the supernatural level to stop it. Why would people invite a curse into their life or allow one to affect them? Because they do not know they are doing it.

If that's the case, why doesn't God do something to help people? He has. He sent Jesus to save the world. When Jesus died on a cross two thousand years ago, he paid the price for Adam's sin — the sin that separated people from God and made the earth a less than perfect place to live. His blood sacrifice opened the door for us to get back to God, back to the good life he intended for us, back to the place of authority to rule the earth that Adam gave Satan when he made a bad choice at mealtime. Thanks to Jesus, a way back to the kingdom of God and all that goes with it has been made available to all people.

Unfortunately, not everyone who has heard about this gift accepts it. Why not? Because they either don't believe Jesus is the Savior of the world or they believe it but don't know what this means to them in terms of fringe benefits. Why don't they believe Jesus saved the world? Or if do they believe it, why don't they use all the advantages that go along with salvation — including the authority to overcome sickness and disease? Because Satan uses deception to keep them in the dark. He blinds unbelievers to the truth of the gospel and deceives believers into thinking that all they got from the cross was a ticket to heaven when they die but no power to improve life on earth before they go.

Why won't God force people to stop living below their privileges? Because God is love and love does not force anyone to do anything. Love opens wide a door and constantly sends a message that love is available. That's what God has been doing since the moment Adam and Eve sinned.

He is like the coach on the sidelines who has given us tactics and strategies to live life successfully. He loves us enough to let us decide for ourselves whether we want to play by the rules he established to protect us on this imperfect planet or whether we want to go our own way. Even when we go our own way, he still sets up an escape route. We either don't recognize it or we reject it.

For instance, a person might eat fried foods every day for forty years and then blame his heart attack on the genes he inherited from his mother. He may never think about biblical teachings warning us not to eat or drink too much. Or he might come down with a disease through no fault of his own but he is unable to believe Psalm 103:3, which says

God heals all our diseases. The choice is simple. We can either fight these curse conditions God's way, or sit back and let Satan slap us around. Let's look at what happens when people don't follow God's plan and allow Satan to take over.

After the Mosaic Law was handed down, God made it abundantly clear that those in covenant relationship with him who disobeyed his commandments would come under a curse (see Deuteronomy 28:15-68). The Bible also says people outside the covenant who disobey the truth and obey unrighteousness are subject to tribulation, anguish, and wrath (Romans 2:8-9). So every curse has a cause (Proverbs 26:2) and can impact believers and non-believers.

Sometimes curses come because of disobedience to God — including the disobedience of an ancestor — or they come because Satan is simply trespassing and no one stopped him. Teachings about generational curses are found in Exodus 20:5 and Exodus 34:6-7, where God warned the Israelites the fathers' iniquities (idol worship and sin) would be visited "upon the children and the children's children to the third and the fourth generation" (Exodus 34:7).

The disciples were no doubt thinking of these passages when they asked Jesus the following question about a man, who had been blind since birth, whom they passed one day while leaving the temple: "'Rabbi, who sinned, this man or his parents, that he was born blind?' Jesus answered, 'Neither this man nor his parents sinned, but that the works of God should be revealed in him' " (John 9:2-3). Jesus then healed the man (John 9:6-7).

The message is clear. This blindness was not caused by the man's sin or his parents' sin. Who knows about his grandparents (the second generation) or great grandparents (the first generation) because the Scriptures are silent on this point. Perhaps they did not sin either. Perhaps this family just tolerated life's troubles (sickness, poverty, mental anguish, etc.) on a fallen planet simply because they did not know what to do about it. They probably saw other blind children in the area and said, "Oh, well. That's just life." Although the cause of this man's blindness is not clear from Scripture, it is clear his healing glorified God and communicated the message that God does not want us sick, handicapped, or diseased.

If you go back a few hundred years in the Bible, there is a story about a member of another Jewish family who decided to fight his sickness supernaturally. His name was Hezekiah. Hezekiah was a descendant of King David and his son Solomon. Solomon started out faithful and wise but ended up carnal and manipulated when he bowed to the wishes of his pagan wives and allowed idol worship in Israel (1 Kings 11:1-6). Just as God had warned, this idol worship plunged a great kingdom into chaos. Generation after generation of bad kings became Judah's legacy and the Jews ultimately ended up back in slavery. Out of seventeen kings from Solomon to Jehoiakim, only three completely did what was right in the eyes of the Lord: Asa (1 Kings 15:9), Hezekiah (2 Kings 18:1-6), and Josiah (2 Kings 21:26).

One day King Hezekiah, who "did what was right in the sight of the Lord, according to all that his father David had done" (2 Kings 18:3), became sick and was near death. Isaiah the prophet went to the palace and told Hezekiah to set his house in order because he was going to die (2 Kings 20:1). But Hezekiah did not take this news lying down. He did not say, "Oh, well. I guess I'm sick because my ancestors were idol worshipers and I'm under a curse." Instead, he prayed and put the Lord in remembrance of how he had walked before him in truth and with a loyal heart (2 Kings 20:2-3). And before Isaiah could even leave the royal residence, the Lord told him to go back and tell Hezekiah his prayer had been heard — he would be healed, and the Lord would add fifteen years to his life and deliver him from his Assyrian enemies (2 Kings 20:4-6).

Was Hezekiah's sickness a result of his ancestors' sins or simply the result of life on an imperfect planet that God used to reveal his works? The Bible does not say. But the important thing to note is that a faith-filled prayer solved the problem regardless of what caused it. That is what a supernatural approach to sickness does. It goes beyond the cause to the solution.

That's what Jesus did when he healed the man blind from birth. We, too, have God-given authority to apply a supernatural solution to a supernatural problem that shows up in the natural world. Once we understand this, we will not do anything to invite sickness and disease — or any other curse for that matter — into our lives or that of our children.

We can also take a good lesson from what happened to a man named Gehazi in the Bible. His story is in 2 Kings 5. Gehazi was a servant to the prophet Elisha. Elisha healed a Syrian army commander named Naaman of leprosy. Naaman wanted to pay Elisha but this man of God refused it.

Gehazi did not think this was a good idea, so he went after Naaman and lied, saying Elisha sent him to get some money for two prophets' sons. Naaman gave Gehazi two talents of silver (equivalent to about $13,000 in 2005 according to online encyclopedia Wikipedia, www.en.wikipedia.org) and two changes of garments. When Gehazi returned to Elisha, Elisha asked where he'd been and Gehazi lied again and said he did not go anywhere. But Elisha knew in his spirit what Gehazi had done and said to him, "'Therefore the leprosy of Naaman shall cling to you and your descendants forever.' And he (Gehazi) went out from his presence leprous, as white as snow." (2 Kings 5:27). Gehazi's greed, lying, and disobedience brought on a curse in the form of a disease.

Disobedience might not always lead to sickness, but we typically end up having some kind of trouble in life when we don't live the way God told us to live. Not because God wants to punish us but because we freely open doors that naturally lead to problems due to our imperfect environment. King Saul, for instance, lost his kingdom to David after he blatantly violated the law of God and made an unlawful sacrifice. (I Samuel 13:9-14). The children of Israel landed under the curse of slavery because of their idol worship. What is the cause of your trouble? Why are you sick? Better yet, why are you sick with the same disease your parent or grandparent had?

Most Christians would deny there has been idol worship in their family history. However, could it have come in the form of food worship handed down recipe by recipe, generation after generation? When you frequently whip up a favorite artery-clogging dish for family gatherings, you could be passing on a gluttonous lifestyle to your children and children's children. You know the drill. Mom heaps more mashed potatoes on her child's plate and says, "Eat some more. You're too skinny. Everybody in this family is fat anyway. Why should you be different?" This attitude, combined with defective genes, could be a recipe for health disasters that impact several members of a family.

Some families have a history of alcoholism, drug addiction, and/or sexual promiscuity. But virtually all families have some kind of food tradition to pass along and it usually does not involve tofu and steamed broccoli. In his book, *The Cost of Being Sick,* Nicholas Webb writes, "Unfortunately, unhealthy lifestyles, like inheritances and heirlooms, can be easily passed down from generation to generation. Many busy parents who value convenience think nothing of sending 'Junior' off to fourth grade with a lunch box full of calorie-laden foodstuffs that fail to meet even minimum dietary guidelines." Just as some physical characteristics may be passed down through families, our cooking and eating habits can also be transferred.

Observe any ethnic group and you will find a food icon. We think of them as symbols of ethnic pride. The Italians have their pastas and breads and cheeses. The French have their rich sauces and delectable pastries. The Mexicans have their tortillas, refried beans, and cheese-laden entrées. And then there are the African Americans. Perhaps no other group worships its food traditions more than black folk in the United States. Fried chicken, chitterlings, macaroni and cheese, potato salad, sweet potato pie, pigs' feet, neck bones, and biscuits and gravy. We like to call it "comfort food." But this comfort food can eventually cause quite a bit of discomfort.

We feast on our favorite dishes to celebrate holidays, birthdays, everyday life, and deaths. It is ironic that we can bury Grandpa after he dies of a heart attack and then go right from the gravesite to the banquet hall and chow down on the very food that probably helped Grandpa to his grave. Few people stop to think that Grandpa might still be with them if he had eaten healthier food. Sometimes family members even brag about how Grandpa "ate whatever he wanted and lived well into his nineties." But no one talks about the angioplasty he had at sixty-five or the quadruple bypass he had at seventy-five, how he was bed-bound from age eighty until he died, or how family members had to quit their jobs to care for him.

I (Christine) noticed this blindness to the problem as shown in the popular 1997 movie *Soul Food*. The story is about an important event that was the anchor for an African-American family living in Chicago. A precocious grandson narrates the story. Every Sunday after church, "Big Mama" and her daughters would prepare a huge family dinner of soul food — complete with the stereotypical overeating "Reverend" in attendance. The family saw this as a lovely tradition that kept them close and helped them deal with life's crises. The opening scene was of a wedding reception. Interestingly enough, the first shot was not of the happy couple but of a dance floor, quickly followed by a long lingering shot of the buffet table — not once, but twice — within the first few minutes of the film. It was filled with roast beef, mashed potatoes, overcooked green beans, and other traditional soul foods.

Later on, it became clear that the very thing designed to bring the family through a crisis actually *caused* the crisis. Big Mama was diagnosed with diabetes, had to have her leg amputated, and subsequently died. Only one line of the movie was devoted to the true cause of her death. When the doctor told the family he would have to cut off one of Big Mama's legs, one of her daughter's said, "Mama, you haven't been watching what you eat." That same daughter helped cook the meals that created Big Mama's health problem. She then turned around and prepared another one after her mother's death to bring the family back together.

This was only a movie. But it is sobering because these scenes are played out at dinner tables and in hospitals around the country every day in America. And it seems to happen very frequently among African-Americans, who tend to be at greater risk for most major diseases such as diabetes and hypertension to name a few. Because of this, some doctors reportedly refer to African-Americans as HONDAs. No, this is not a reference to the Japanese automobile. It is an acronym describing the typical health problems seen among this ethnic group. It stands for: Hypertension, Obesity, Nutritionally Deficient, Diabetic, and Arthritic.

Other ethnic groups have their higher risk diseases too. But somehow, we just don't get it. We don't get it when we get sick. We don't get it when our loved ones die. We don't get it even though the younger generation is getting sicker and sicker right before our very eyes — struck down by diseases not heard of among children years ago, at least not in such alarming numbers.

Television actor John Ritter died September 12, 2003, of a heart condition called aortic dissection. He was fifty-four years old. WebMD.com describes this condition as "an abnormal separation of tissues within the walls of the aorta" that can be caused by high blood pressure, chest injury, or a family history of aortic dissection. The media were quick to report Ritter's father had died of a heart attack in 1974 at age sixty-seven. Did John Ritter die of this condition because of global imperfection, a generational curse, or a clash between defective genes and a poor diet? The reporters did not comment on why they thought both this father and son died from heart-related conditions. They probably just considered it the normal course of life. Wouldn't it have been great if they had reported this does not have to happen to John's children? Instead, in a December 1, 2003, special edition of *U.S. News & World Report* there was a story about the discovery of a so-called "heart attack gene."

The last thing we need is a report of this kind to make us think we cannot do anything about our own health. Even if there is such a gene, we do not have to allow it to attack. Stories like this do not inspire hope. They inspire fear. They make people think it's just going to happen anyway in their family so why try to fight it. Just eat what you want and don't worry about it.

But lifestyle does matter and generational lifestyles have more to do with our current lives than we care to think. On the natural level, think about your family's health history. Are there any particular diseases that seem to land in your family tree often? Are there some common lifestyles associated with these diseases? Eating pork twice a day? Eating mostly fried foods? Passing up the vegetables for the starches and sweets?

Since many people do not have huge financial legacies to pass on to their descendants, the least they can do is pass along the wisdom to stay healthy so they can be about God's business. "It" does not have to run in the family. Despite your situation and your ancestors' genes or lifestyles, you can take authority over "it," run it out of the family, and teach your children and your children's children to do likewise.

Chapter Summary

1. Too many people not only expect to get the sicknesses and diseases that have historically run in their families, but they also accept them as just a normal part of life.
2. On the natural level, most chronic conditions occur when the genes we inherit from our ancestors interact with environmental factors that can be controlled, such as smoking and poor dietary habits.
3. Spiritually, sickness and disease can occur because it is invited by disobeying God or is allowed when we fail to exercise the authority God gave us to overcome it.
4. Too many families pass on unhealthy eating traditions to their children. These strongholds need to be broken if they rise to the level of idol worship.

Kristy Dotson & Christine Tennon

Story from the Front Lines...

Mother Overcomes Obesity and Trains Up Child

Heather Caliare was celebrating her first Christmas with her husband. He told her to go out and buy herself something nice. At 250 pounds she thought she was about a size eighteen, but while trying on outfits, she discovered even a size twenty was too small.

"I had to go into a size 22," Heather says.

Horrified, she went home and told her husband, "We've got to do something!" So she decided to change. She prayed, changed her eating habits, and began to exercise regularly.

Heather lost a lot of weight and ended up a size 9/10. As she puts it, "You cannot do it without faith."

Heather comes from a family in which obesity and obesity-related disease is common. When Heather was four years old, her mother died of cancer, as did a favorite uncle. She went to live with an aunt. Five years later, that aunt died of cancer. In fifth grade, Heather was 5'8" and a size fourteen.

"You can imagine how it was in school," Heather says. "In gym class, people would say things like, 'Get up, Big Mama.' They'd laugh at me and I'll never forget that."

Heather says she grew up in a rural area where the food was very unhealthy. She says the cooks in her family would actually pour grease used to fry other foods into the vegetables when they cooked them.

When Heather became pregnant, she vowed her child would have a different life. She says, "I was a fat child and I will do everything to keep my child from being fat. People are so cruel." After the baby was born, Heather picked up a little weight but continued her exercise regimen and a healthy diet of whole foods. She and her husband are also focusing on the proper foods for their son.

Heather told her husband, "I will not have my child grow up heavy because I know how kids are. I don't even want my child to know what a McDonald's sandwich is."

She has made a lot of changes. "We don't eat beef or pork. We eat chicken and fish — salmon only," she says. "I told my husband, if we teach our son now the things we were supposed to be taught, he'll grow up healthy and won't have to worry about sickness or diseases. We will not have him grow up the way I did."

Chapter Five

Surrounded by the Enemy

It isn't a shortage of food that causes mass starvation, nor too much food that causes mass obesity. Our problems belong not to food itself, as I had assumed all those years, but to the attitudes people have about food and how those attitudes are influenced and manipulated.
~ Paul A. Stitt, Beating the Food Giants

It's Monday morning and you've overslept! "What's up with this alarm clock?" you yell. You rush around and finally get the kids off to school with lunch money and no breakfast. Then you check the refrigerator to see what you can brown bag for your midday meal. Darn! It's slim pickings. No leftovers from Sunday dinner. You had take-out from KFC and your family barely left the chicken bones.

Oh, well, I'll just grab something at work, you decide as you rush out the door.

This was supposed to be your week for exercising but the bike you bought two months ago is still in the box. You dropped your gym membership six months back. Since you just could not find the time to go, it did not make sense to keep paying those high fees.

But I'll do better when I get more time, you tell yourself on the drive to work.

You figure the best way to do this "weight-loss thing" is to start small. So instead of taking the escalator in your building to the lobby level, you resolve to take the stairs. At least that's something. Besides, you feel pretty confident about being able to lose a lot of weight on a low carb diet. Last time you were too stressed out to stick to it. But you are determined to do it for real this time without cheating.

Now that you have a plan, you feel better and turn on the car radio as you sit on the freeway headed to your downtown job. The traffic report comes on. You groan inwardly, "Man! It's a parking lot this morning! I should have grabbed a snack — one of those raspberry breakfast bars the kids like so much." You reach for an inspirational music CD. Before you put it in, a commercial comes on for "Gooey Yummy" cinnamon rolls. Your mouth waters as you think, *I love those things. Too bad the only places that sell them are in the far north suburbs.* You hastily scribble a note to pick up some on the weekend.

Before going into your downtown office building, you take a detour to the bakery next door. Your favorite raspberry and cream cheese Danish is on sale. You buy two — one for now, the other for your afternoon break. Since you are already late, you stop and buy a double chocolate mocha Frappuccino. Finally, you plop down at your desk at 8:20 a.m. A co-worker stops by and asks you to sign a birthday card for Susie, another employee in your department. She also whispers, "We're gonna have cake for her in the break room at ten." You nod, whip out the Danish, gulp down the coffee and start returning telephone calls.

At ten o'clock, the crowd gathers in the break room to celebrate another year in Susie's life. You join them out of peer pressure. You don't really like Susie. But, you like her cake. German chocolate is your favorite. So you take a "small slice," wrap it up and return to your desk. You say to yourself, "I'll take it home and have it after dinner since I already had the Danish."

Lunchtime rolls around. As you stretch at your desk and contemplate what you will eat, your phone rings. After noticing the caller's phone number, you reluctantly answer as you lament to yourself, *Oh, great, it's the office cheerleader!* She tells you in a tone much too chipper for your current mood, "The gang is taking Susie out for her birthday. We're going for Mexican food at El Mercado's. It's Susie's favorite. Meet us there at 12:15." You thought about making an excuse for not going, but everybody at work always makes such a big deal if an employee misses a co-worker's milestone event. Besides, the boss was picking up the tab.

Only a crazy person passes up a free lunch! you think.

You meet "the gang" at 12:15 sharp. The waitress brings salsa and chips. Somebody orders nachos and quesadillas as appetizers. The platters are passed around and you help yourself. For your entrée, you order the beef burrito with refried beans, rice, and a diet cola. The waiter brings Susie the obligatory cupcake with a candle on top. You all sing "Happy Birthday" to her and go back to work bloated and sluggish.

Later that afternoon, when you go on break, you grab your other Danish and have it with another diet cola. An hour later, your boss sends an e-mail reminding everyone that the Girl Scout cookies they ordered are in. You had bought seven boxes. Your kids love them and they keep in the freezer for a long time. Driving home in horrendous traffic, you break out a box of the cookies. By the time you get home an hour later, you've eaten half of them and applaud your self-restraint.

At home that evening, your children want pizza. You order two — one large supreme with all of the ingredients and one large pepperoni. There were no leftovers. That slice of Susie's cake you brought home was your dessert. By the time the late news comes on, you have heartburn. You take some over-the-counter medicine for it and vow never to eat pizza so late again. You nod off to sleep on the sofa before the weather comes on. At midnight you wake up and drag yourself to bed.

It's Tuesday. Back at work, you go through your same breakfast routine except you get a chocolate chip muffin instead of the Danish. There are no birthdays today, but one of your business vendors left some caramel popcorn at the front desk. Someone put it in a bowl in the break room with a sign that says, "Help yourself." You take a few nibbles when you go for your mid-morning break and wash it down with coffee. On the way back to your desk, a co-worker stops you in the hall. He is selling candy to raise money for his son's school band. You buy two bars to help the worthy cause.

At lunchtime, you glance at the clock, look at the ever-increasing pile of work on your desk and decide to grab a salad from the place next door and rush back to work.

Mmmmm. It looks fresh today, you think as you peruse the salad bar. *I'll just get a small one with lite dressing.*

As you navigate the bar, you start with iceberg lettuce, add a little spinach for "health," and then toss in some cheddar cheese, tomatoes, and mushrooms. The croutons beckon so you add a few for flavor.

"Ooohhh! They have the little fried chicken strips today. Boy, I love those things on salads," you say out loud. You add six to the top of your "small" salad.

Now for the dressing. You reach for the "Lite" brand to balance things out. But the guy behind you says, "I'd get the blue cheese if I were you. It tastes so much better on top of the chicken strips."

You nod in agreement and say, "But the 'Lite' looks so much better around my waist."

He replies, "Ah, come on. You don't have anything to worry about. Besides, I always tell myself I can work it off later, so you can, too."

You shrug and say, "You're right. Anyway, this little bit won't kill me." At the checkout counter, you grab a diet cola, saltine crackers, and a box of animal cookies.

Back at your desk, you hurriedly eat while glancing over your work. At two o'clock, you decide to take a break. You feel kind of sleepy and think, *I need a pick me up.*

Walking through the break room, you stop by the snack machine. "Oh, neat, they've added those new potato chips I saw on TV the other night," you say to yourself. Seventy-five cents later, you are munching the chips, washing them down with another diet cola.

On the way back to your desk, you stop and chat with a co-worker. He has a dish of chocolate kisses on his desk. You grab a few. Twenty minutes later, you feel a bit more energetic. But an hour later, you feel that lull again. You cannot wait to get home.

What will we do for dinner tonight? you wonder. On the way home, you plan your menu. Once there, you cook up some spaghetti and meatballs with French bread and salad. Ice cream is on hand for dessert.

Two weeks later, you go on vacation. It is a cruise complete with round-the-clock meal service. You have your choice of a breakfast buffet or a sit-down meal with waiters in white jackets standing by to make your every food wish come true. French toast? No problem. With whipped cream and chocolate chips? Coming right up. Out by the pool, burgers, pizza, and hot dogs are plentiful. Soft drinks, coffee, and tea are free, but water is $2.25 a bottle. In the spa, there is fruit and some energy bars loaded with sugar. On shore excursions, lunch at a local restaurant is included with the ground transportation. A key part of the tours is to make sure everyone gets back in time for their scheduled dinner seatings.

One night as you read the ship's dinner menu, you think, *Boy, this stuff should come with a free angioplasty.* Surf and turf, pastas in heavy creams, salads in creamy dressings, exotic appetizers wrapped in high-fat, baskets of bread with real butter, and crème brûlée, Bananas Foster, or Baked Alaska for dessert. You vow each night to keep it lean and clean. But when the waiter announces the night's menu in that wonderful Romanian accent, you smile benignly and order something for all five courses. You just cannot bring yourself to hurt his feelings — he seems so sad when anyone tries to forego a course. It is a vacation and everyone goes a little overboard with food on vacation, you reason. It's expected.

At church a month later, you attend an evening volunteer meeting with the children's Sunday school staff. They serve chicken tenders, with cookies for dessert. You brought a salad but the lady sitting next to you offers you three of the tenders.

"They'll be good on that salad," she says with a lovely "I'm trying to be a good Christian sister" smile on her face.

A week later, your neighbor says she has started selling *Mary Kay* cosmetics and invites you to a party. She serves nachos, pigs in a blanket, and cake with pink frosting. There are some leftovers and you stay to help clean up. She sends half of the remaining food home with you, saying, "You can take it to work tomorrow for lunch. That way you won't have to buy anything downtown."

On the way home, you stop at the mall to pick up some sneakers for your son. You park near the entrance to the food court. All of your favorites are there — McDonald's,

Taco Bell, Mrs. Fields Cookies, and every other precursor to indigestion and thunder thighs you can wrap your lips around.

And so it continues, day after day, week after week, year after year. The foods you love and that hate your body are everywhere. And everywhere you turn you get ample encouragement to eat them to your heart's content. Family, friends, strangers, and billboards urge you on.

Even your doctor gives you a little nudge in the same direction. "Moderation," he says, "is the key. You can't give up everything. Have a little treat every now and then but watch the fat and count your calories." For that wealth of nutritional advice, you paid your $20 HMO co-pay, stopped at the grocery store on the way home, picked up some hot wings, and promptly forgot what the doctor said.

One day you decide to start a new eating plan and stick to it. You come up with your own version of the low-carb diet craze. You feel better and you lose weight. But at work, everybody gives you grief.

"Ah, come on! Live a little. You're young," they say. "Why would you give up bagels and cream cheese? And coffee? You *must* be sick. How can you get your morning started without it? Our whole office runs on this stuff!"

On and on it goes. At work, at social events, at church! Eat this. Eat that. Eat, eat, eat! And then your boss plans an out of town business meeting — complete with catered luncheons and lavish dinners. Feeling doomed, you throw up both your hands and indulge!

Do you think Eve felt this way in the Garden of Eden when she had her little repartee with Satan disguised as a serpent? Today, Satan's proxies are still offering us a form of forbidden fruit and urging us to eat to our heart's destruction. We end up consuming food that damages our cells and turns our bodies into hosts for debilitating diseases. Taste overcomes willpower and the path to slow suicide becomes broader and broader. Yet nothing really changes. Instead of poor eating habits dying, people are dying before their appointed times. Chalk up another one for the enemy.

Just look at the person in the scenario above. She apparently spent as much time at work snacking as working. I (Christine) inventoried the snack machines at my workplace and realized they are nothing but big boxes of sugar and salt. I actually made a list of the contents. There were six different candies (Snickers, M&M's peanut, M&M's plain, Payday, Reese's Fast Break, and Reese's Pieces), fourteen snack chips and popcorns (Doritos 1¾ oz., Doritos 1 oz., Cheetos Crunchy, Cheetos Flamin' Hot, Ruffles, Lays, Jays Hot Stuff, Cheddar Fries, Cheetos Puffs, O-Ke-Doke Popcorn, Bugles, Sunchips

Harvest Cheddar, Fritos Cheddar Ranch, and Popz Microwave Popcorn), four cookie choices (Lorna Doones, chocolate sandwich cream cookies, Chips Ahoy, and boysenberry shortbread cookies), and two pastries (Hostess Apple Fruit Pie and pineapple cheese Danish). That machine saw a lot of business. Employees were thrilled when a new machine was installed that could change a one-dollar bill.

I (Kristy) worked for a processed foods company that brought the snacks to the employees. So getting a sugar rush each day was easy. Every day at ten a.m. and two p.m., a "dessert cart" was rolled around the floor so employees did not have to go downstairs for snacks. How convenient!

Most workplaces are very structured. People eat out of boredom or to relieve stress. In January 2004, a survey by the American Association of Working People showed 89 percent of those polled snacked during the workday and more than half of them ate things like chips, candy, doughnuts, and cookies.

But the biggest motivation to eat and eat is our culture. Food is the axis around which our lives revolve. And most of the food so readily available to us is designed for two purposes: to tickle our taste buds so we will want more and to generate profits for the food manufacturers. There is nothing wrong with either motive except that they are given priority over good nutrition. Take a look around. The evidence is everywhere.

Pick up the newspaper on any given Sunday. Inside, you will find an overabundance of advertisements — many of them for food items. After I (Christine) reviewed these circulars one Sunday morning it suddenly struck me that most of the food marketed by retailers can undermine good health if these items hold a prominent place in our diets. But here is the real irony: the newspaper also contained ads for items that can ease symptoms brought on by eating too much of the food being marketed.

One Sunday, a major pharmacy chain had among its sale items at least eight different candy bars — yummy sweet concoctions of chocolate, caramel, peanuts, almonds, and several other ingredients you need a Ph.D. to pronounce. Those additives with the mile-long names are there to make sure your goodies have a long shelf life. This spells convenience for the consumer, capital for the manufacturing company, and possibly cancer for your cells. Also included were ads for a well-loved cookie sprinkled with chocolate chips, highly processed figs wrapped in a soft cookie, that famous dark chocolate sweet treat that tempts you to eat the white creamy middle first, bread that makes you wonder, chips of which you can't eat just one, beef slathered with tomato sauce in a can, canned chili, and sodas, coffee, and whole milk to wash it all down.

Any one of the above food items could generate some serious gastrointestinal disturbances — heartburn, indigestion, and the like. But this chain had all the bases covered in the customer-friendly fashion Americans have come to expect. Conveniently included in its Sunday circular were also palliatives to stifle that gurgling stomach, soothe that burning chest, ease that headache, and deal with the extra weight the cookies, chips, and chili add to your body. Among these remedies were Pepcid AC (with the slogan "relieves heartburn due to acid indigestion"), Advil, Aleve, Maalox, Tylenol Arthritis, Zantac 75 ("prevents and relieves heartburn associated with acid indigestion and sour stomach"), Tums, Prilosec OTC ("treats frequent heartburn"), Slim-Fast, Starch Away, Stacker ("world's strongest fat burner"), One-A-Day WeightSmart, Diabaid (antifungal foot bath and other body products), and the Lumiscope Blood Pressure Monitor.

Looking through some newspaper coupons one day, I (Christine) noticed most of the coupons were for items we do not need — fudge cookies, sugar-laden breakfast bars and cereals, juices with multiple processed sweeteners, cheesy pastas, ice creams, French onion dips, biscuits, pizza, taco kits, and frozen dinners preserved with far more sodium than any person needs. While running an errand I saw a sign at a fast food restaurant advertising burgers at two for three dollars. A few days later it read "Burgers: 2 for $2.22." It was cheap. It was fast. It was tasty. That is a hard combination to beat in today's time-crunched society. It is in the face of this kind of commercial bombardment that we have to make wise decisions about what to eat. But temptation is ever before us.

I (Christine) went to the grocery store to pick up a few items one night. I was in a hurry and frankly did not have world health issues on my mind at the time. A few minutes after I walked in the store, I felt a tug on my psyche urging me to look around. So I stopped and scanned the store. I thought, *Even the outside aisles are not safe!* I had always heard shopping the outside aisles of the grocery store ensures healthier food choices. But this is not always true in today's food market. To confirm my initial impression, I strolled the outside aisles with a notepad. Here is what I saw.

On the aisle of the store's western wall, the produce section was on the left. On the right side was every variety of cheese you could imagine: Cheddar, goat, Gorgonzola, Edam, Colby jack, Swiss, Parmesan, mozzarella, feta, and American, to name a few. My eye was also drawn to party trays with pepperoni, salami, beef sticks and more cheese, fettuccine, ravioli, macaroni salad, cold cuts, pizza, hot wings, egg rolls, ham, chicken nuggets, bacon, cold cuts, hot dogs, and smoked sausage. At the end of the western aisle, there was a doughnut stand — chocolate sprinkled, glazed, cream-filled, devil's food, etc.

At that point, the aisle for the northern wall of the store began. I saw a glass case on the left containing bagels and more doughnuts. Next to it were shelves containing pound cakes, coffee cakes, cookies, fudge cake, apple pies, chess pies, chocolate cream pies, more doughnuts, muffins, croissants, cheesecake, éclairs, carrot cake, strawberry cake, and a chocolate torte. (I still was shopping just the outside aisle!) On my right were fruit juice, cookies, more doughnuts, ice cream cakes, and a display full of candy bars.

Farther down on my left was the deli section. I smelled the aroma of fried food. My nose did not deceive me. Encased in glass were fried chicken, "fresh" hot wings, and fried potatoes. Next to it was the potato salad, macaroni salad, mini chicken corn dogs, cheese-bacon baked potatoes, meatloaf, shrimp salad, beef tamales, pastrami, ham, bologna, hog's headcheese, corned beef, London broil, and more cheese.

Continuing my journey, I came upon the meat and seafood section — catfish fillets, catfish nuggets, small catfish, shrimp, crab legs, pot roast, filet mignon, chicken, ground beef, ground turkey, smoked turkey, etc. Opposite the meat counter were potato chips, soft drinks (orange, grape, peach, root beer, colas, lemon-limes, cherry flavored, etc.), pork cracklins, pork skins, cheese curls, and ice cream cakes ("Buy 1, get 1 free"). At the front of the store, the aisle spanning the southern wall had orange juice concentrates, honey buns, raisin cakes, marshmallow pies, oatmeal cream pies, nutty bars, Atkins low carb foods (shakes, chocolate cream bars, breakfast bars), ice cream, cornbread, more potato chips, corn chips, pretzels, more cheese curls, more sodas, tortillas, and coffee. As this was late January, approaching the checkout stand I saw a huge "Super Bowl Party" display containing the usual munchies.

Once in line to pay for my items, my eyes went to the racks by the cash registers. A variety of cookies were in easy reach as were several candy bars, some "3 for 96¢" and others with packaging boasting "most nuts ever" or "packed with more nuts." (I won't mention the magazines and tabloids — that is a subject for a different book!) While I waited to pay, I could not help but notice over 50 percent of the people in line were overweight or obese. Three of the four checkout clerks were overweight or obese.

I had walked to the store. It was only three blocks. On my way home I noticed there were three pizza restaurants and a chicken restaurant in that three-block area. The chicken place advertised "7 Hot Wings $2.99" and "20-piece Hot BBQ Wings $7.99." One pizza place had a sign that read "Pepperoni Pizza $4.49."

What I saw felt like sensory overload. Everything I glimpsed appealed to the flesh and turned my thoughts to my body — what looked good to eat, what tasted good. All this after a short hike to the grocery store! The magnitude of the challenge to eat well was brought home to me afresh. I suddenly felt overwhelmed and prayed, *Lord, how can we overcome this? Please show us how!*

I (Christine) felt the same way one day when I came home from work and there was a chicken leg hanging on my mailbox. It was paper, of course, but a pretty good replica of the real thing. The restaurant was advertising its "Martin Luther King, Jr. Day Special."

And then there is television, that society-changing invention that former Federal Communications Commission Chairman Newton Minow called a "vast wasteland." Every few minutes or so — unless we are watching a commercial-free channel — this little box ushers a food temptation (not to mention others enticements) into our homes. Perhaps I should say multiple rooms of our homes. There is usually a big box in the living area and smaller boxes in each bedroom.

One night I (Christine) saw back-to-back commercials about food. The first featured ice cream, candy bars, and other sweet treats that could supposedly "help you lose weight." It was followed by ads for Kool-Aid and a butter substitute. Then came the ad encouraging people to befriend their pharmacists. I even saw one macaroni and cheese commercial where the announcer bragged about how the portions had been enlarged to accommodate growing teenagers. Just what we need: more starchy cheesy food to help our already obese children grow bigger and sicker.

The worst are the ads for foods that sound healthy but omit the not-so-healthy fine print. Take this one television commercial that promoted a fruit spread claiming its contents — apricots, strawberries, and blueberries — were "picked at the peak of perfection." When you read the ingredient listing, you see the contents, in order of prominence, are high fructose corn syrup, sugar, and a whole host of things you need a science degree to pronounce. It makes you wonder what fruit was picked from an orchard as opposed to those created by a scientist in a laboratory.

One day I (Christine) picked up my Sunday newspaper and out fell a packet of French vanilla cappuccino. The labeling was designed to entice. It read, "Sip into something decadent!"

Even the piece of plastic used to cover my dry cleaning occasionally pushes food. One day I noticed an ad for a popular pizza chain was embossed on it that read, "Make the next stop your grocer's freezer. Enjoy one of our unique pizzas at home." I thought, *This bombardment is never-ending!*

I can't open my front door, pick up my dry cleaning, turn on the TV or radio, or drive down the street past a billboard without having food shoved at me. Correction: without having the *unhealthiest* food shoved at me.

Let's face it. Nutritionally bankrupt food is at our fingertips no matter where we go. Maybe you have tried to stop eating this stuff, but it is hard to do. Despite your vows and pledges to give it up, these foods just always seem to be present at home, at work, at church, and at social events. Of course, you have a responsibility not to overeat them. But how do you carry out that responsibility? Announce another diet and then "cheat" behind the scenes? No. Don't do that. Instead, take heart from this story in 2 Kings.

The Syrian army surrounded the city of Dothan where the Hebrew prophet Elisha was living. The king of Syria wanted to get rid of Elisha because he was undermining his country's war effort against Israel. Every time Syria planned to attack Israel, it was supernaturally revealed to Elisha and he would warn the king of Israel. So acting on the king's orders, the Syrian army went off to Dothan to find Elisha.

> *Therefore he sent horses and chariots and a great army there, and they came by night and surrounded the city. And when the servant of the man of God arose early and went out, there was an army, surrounding the city with horses and chariots. And his servant said to him, "Alas, my master! What shall we do?" So he answered, "Do not fear, for those who are with us are more than those who are with them." And Elisha prayed, and said, "Lord, I pray, open his eyes that he may see." Then the Lord opened the eyes of the young man, and he saw. And behold, the mountain was full of horses and chariots of fire all around Elisha. So when the Syrians came down to him, Elisha prayed to the Lord, and said, "Strike this people, I pray, with blindness." And He struck them with blindness according to the word of Elisha.*
> *~ 2 Kings 6:14-18*

If God can deliver Elisha from the hand of a vicious army, he can certainly deliver you from foods that will slowly turn on you and destroy your health. This will not happen, however, until you take off the blinders and begin to see many foods in the marketplace as weapons poised against you. So stay on the alert. Put on your spiritual dietary armor and begin defending your physical temple each time you pick up your fork.

Chapter Summary

1. Food that does not nourish the body always seems to be more available than nutritious food.
2. Consumers are often encouraged by friends, family, co-workers, strangers and the mass media to eat nutritionally bankrupt food.
3. A key strategy in the battle for health is to recognize unhealthy foods and resist the temptation to eat them day by day, meal by meal.

Chapter Six

The Motive Behind the Meal

For human beings, eating has never been a simple matter. To a frog snagging a fly or a pelican nabbing a fish, food is fuel and nothing more. To a human, the ritual of eating – the act of pulling up and tucking in, or passing around and helping oneself – is one of the most primal of shared activities.
~ Jeffrey Kluger, Why We Eat – Time, June 7, 2004

Do you eat when you are not hungry? If so, why? Eating for reasons other than hunger seems to be quite common these days. But this was not always so. During the hunter-gatherer period of human history, people only ate enough food to keep from starving to death. The males went out to hunt wild game and feed their tribes. They risked life and limb to bring meat to the table. They didn't care whether it was fried, sautéed, barbequed, or drowned in salt and spices. They just wanted to stay strong enough to fight off warring tribes and survive harsh weather conditions.

This motive for eating did not change very much during the agricultural age. People worked the land and grew crops. Their reasons were simple: they needed to provide food and a source of income for their families. They ate to survive. As with the hunter-gatherers, their main goal was to have enough food to keep from starving to death. In those days, dying from lack of food was just one drought away.

The same is true of Bible times. Famine was a frequent theme in the Old Testament. Stories about people contending with a lack of food can be found in the following passages: Abram in Canaan, Genesis 12:10; Isaac in Canaan, Genesis 26:1; Joseph in Egypt, Genesis 41:54; Jacob in Canaan, Genesis 41:56; Bethlehem famine, Ruth 1:1; Famine in David's day, 2 Samuel 21:1; Elisha and the famine in Gilgal, 2 Kings 4:38; Samaria famine so severe a woman boiled her son and ate him, 2 Kings 6:25-29; famine that impacted Elijah and the widow of Zaraphath, 1 Kings 17:1-24; and the Jerusalem famine, 2 Kings 25:3.

Today, Americans live in what is considered a "land of plenty" where many people have enough to eat. So our food problems are often quite different from those faced by people in ancient times or our ancestors of a few generations ago. The vast majority of Americans usually can manage to get enough food to keep from starving. For the most part, our challenge is not lack of food but the kind of food we eat and why we eat it.

Everyone knows, at least in theory, that healthy eating is good for the body. However, it seems that is not why many people eat. Some eat for fun versus fuel. Or they eat to reward or "treat" themselves. When people look at a buffet table full of food and say, "Oh that looks good!" they are not commenting on how the goodies will help their cells rebuild and resist disease or help the heart pump blood through their bodies. They are commenting on the taste of the food, and its ability to tickle their tongue and satisfy their hunger for something they "like" to eat.

When I (Christine) was a felony prosecutor, one of my favorite things to do after a hard day of prosecuting criminals was to swing by a French bread bakery and get myself a "treat" for my psyche — not my body. The needs of my internal organs were the last thing on my mind. For some people, a vodka martini would do the trick. But food was my balm. It eased my troubled mind and helped me cope, or so I thought, with the challenges of modern work life. I felt it was the least I could do for myself. After all, I was keeping the community safe from robbers, rapists, and murderers! But I was not keeping my body safe from disease. I was winning the battle in the courtroom and losing the fight for my own health.

What my body needed was irrelevant to me at that time. It could fend for itself as far as my head was concerned. My emotional state needed nurturing and if that meant going a week without a green leafy vegetable, then so be it. I had to eat away the stress of the job. I had to eat away the depression over being divorced and broke. I had to eat away my frustration with family, the dry cleaner, rude drivers on the freeway, the alarm clock, the birds chirping at my window each morning, chipped nail polish, torn hosiery, etc.

So my reason for eating was no longer physical survival. It was emotional survival. Food became my fix. I never analyzed my mental needs beyond finding the next food treat to calm myself down. Once this way of thinking was set, my flesh fell in line with it. If my eyes saw cheesecake and my brain said, "That will make you feel better," I ate cheesecake. If my brain said, "A second slice won't hurt. You deserve it. You've been good all day," then I ate a second piece. Later, my mind would turn on me and I'd think, *I feel sick. I should not have eaten all that cheesecake. I'm going to get fat and have to buy new clothes. I'll end up fat and broke.*

My crazy thoughts about food got plenty of reinforcement. At every party or social event, other guests would tell me, "Eat up. Taste it. Try it. Have some more. You deserve it. You're not fat." When I was a child, I remember hearing adults tell children who would not eat their meals, "You'd better eat this food and not waste it. Children in India are starving." Or I would hear TV moms tell their kids, "Eat your vegetables. You're a growing boy (or girl). It's good for you." Nowadays, people tell us to eat something only because it tastes good. The elderly and sick usually are the only ones who are told they must eat to keep up their strength. Oddly enough, I never have heard of anyone being told this *before* they get sick.

Webster defines "strength" as "power of resisting attack, impregnability; capacity for exertion or endurance; power to resist force; solidity, toughness; a strong attribute or inherent asset; a degree of potency of effect." Does the food you eat consistently do this for your body? Better yet, are you even thinking about wanting your food to do this for your body when you are choosing your food? For most folks, their only thought is, *Boy, I hope this tastes as good as it looks.* What would happen if before every meal we would ask ourselves, "Will eating this keep my cells strong and my organs working properly?" We would probably pass up some of the dead stuff that always seems to be around for us to munch on.

Years ago, there was not as much health and nutrition information available as there is today. So we don't have much of an excuse these days for not eating healthier food. A multi-billion dollar industry screams at us on every corner about "proper nutrition." Go to your local bookstore. There is a whole section devoted to this subject. Several celebrities have a book, DVD, and/or an opinion on how to be healthy. You probably own some of their products or a piece of exercise equipment they designed or endorsed. But none of it will do you any good until you understand why you eat the way you do and begin to apply biblical wisdom to this area of your life.

Jane's husband dumped her for one of her friends. So, she replaced him with apple pie over and over again. The weight gain did not matter. Neither did the shortness of breath she started to experience. She thought, *I don't need to be thin and bubbly. I'm thirty-six years old and manless and will no doubt stay that way forever.* So eating was her consolation. Perhaps Isaiah 54:5-6 could have helped. It says, "'For your Maker is your husband, the Lord of hosts is His name; And your redeemer is the Holy One of Israel; He is called the God of the whole earth. For the Lord has called you like a woman forsaken and grieved in spirit, like a youthful wife when you were refused,' says your God."

Bill's archenemy at work got the promotion Bill had wanted even though Bill was better qualified. So he indulged himself with his favorite food — beef enchiladas and Haagen-Dazs ice cream — for weeks. When he developed digestive problems, Bill went to the doctor and got a prescription. It helped his stomach so he kept wolfing down the enchiladas to soothe his bruised ego. The ice cream calmed his anger. But the Bible has a better salve for the wounded spirit. Proverbs 18:16 says, "A man's gift makes room for him, and brings him before great men." Proverbs 22:29 says, "Do you see a man who excels in his work? He will stand before kings."

Ephron ate for company. He was alone in a new city after a job transfer. He had no family or friends there. So at the end of long workdays, he'd call a little Italian restaurant near his apartment and order dinner. The chef there made the best fettuccine Alfredo Ephron had ever tasted. And the tiramisu was to die for! And he almost did. A year into the job, Ephron had a heart attack. Now that he has had a quadruple bypass, he only eats at that restaurant once a week. But he's still lonely. Yet in the Bible, God tells us, "I will never leave you nor forsake you" (Hebrew 13:5) and Jesus said he will be with us "always, even to the end of the age" (Matthew 28:20). Proverbs 18:24 says, "A man who has friends must himself be friendly, but there is a friend who sticks closer than a brother."

Allison ate to take her mind off her wayward daughter. The girl was eighteen and living with a thirty-two-year-old man who had her hooked on cocaine. She would not even take Allison's telephone calls. But the local pizzeria would. In fact, they were on a first-name basis with Allison. They knew her order by heart: one large sausage pizza with extra cheese. But Jesus came "to heal the broken hearted" and "proclaim liberty to the captives" (Luke 4:18). The story of the prodigal son in Luke 15 beautifully illustrates this promise and still inspires hope in parents 2,000 years later.

On and on the stories go. Everybody has one. Here is a particularly sad example. "Jim" was glad to be home after his quadruple bypass surgery. "Hospital food was for the birds," he said. "It did not taste good. Those cooks just did not know how to properly season food. Bland, bland, bland!" But the doctor's instructions for his diet were clear: no fried foods, no pork, no salt, no fatty foods; plenty of fresh vegetables and fruit. Yet, as a welcome home treat, his wife prepared him pork neck bones and spaghetti. And so Jim continued to eat poorly — fried chicken, fried catfish, pork bacon, pigs' feet, etc.

Leukemia and other health problems (high blood pressure, diabetes, and so on) got the better of Jim and he eventually died. But he got to eat his favorite foods right up to the end. Was he eating to live or eating to die? Was he eating to maintain his freshly unclogged arteries? Did his family feed him in a way that would restore his health and keep his body functioning as God intended? Or did they feed that place in him that had an overwhelming yearning for forbidden food — food that would destroy the doctor's surgical handiwork and send Jim right back to death's door and eventually through it? Did they help him slowly but surely kill himself, arguably before his time?

Why would a person in a health crisis disobey his or her doctor's dietary orders? What power is so strong that it would make such a rational and gifted person overlook the connection between what he ate, the quality of his health, and his ability to carry out his Christian responsibilities well beyond the age of 66? It is the power of thought.

What we think determines what we do. If your mind says, "Eat more fried chicken," your mouth will oblige because our thought life drives our appetites. So when it comes to food and physical health, we are what we think *and* what we eat. But if we control the mind, we can control our eating. How do we control the mind? Renew it. The apostle Paul said it this way in his letter to the Romans:

> *I beseech you therefore, brethren, by the mercies of God, that you present your bodies a living sacrifice, holy acceptable to God, which is your reasonable service. And do not be conformed to this world, but be transformed by the renewing of your mind, that you may prove what is that good and acceptable and perfect will of God.*
> *~ Romans 12:1-2*

Each day you have a choice to make about what food you put into your body. Will you feed your cells or feed your emotions? If your mind tells you to feed your body toxic food early and often, tell it to shut up. Tell it you are a "living sacrifice" and that you have a renewed mind. In fact, the Bible says, "we have the mind of Christ" (1 Corinthians 2:16). The mind of Christ proves what is that good and "acceptable and perfect will of God." Eating ourselves into an early grave is not his perfect will. Remember, a mind un-renewed to God's way of living is a terrible thing to obey.

Keep your guard up because your flesh will test you. It does not want your mind renewed or your body to be a living sacrifice to God. I heard Pastor Mike Hayes of Covenant Church in Carrollton, Texas, say we should not be shocked by the cravings of the flesh. As he put it, "The flesh has no investment in eternity." Hayes said the flesh knows it usually has about seventy years on this planet to try to do whatever it wants and then goes back to the dust.

Since the flesh has no interest in the things of God, we have to bring it into submission to his will. So if we do not tell our bodies what to do, instead of it telling us what to do, we will end up missing our destiny or have it prematurely interrupted by sickness, disease, and death. As Joyce Meyer says in her book, *Battlefield of the Mind*, "Right thinking is vital to victorious living."

Back in the late 1800s some very smart people tried to address the issue of eating and spirituality. Author Michelle Stacey mentions this in her book, *Consumed: Why Americans Love, Hate and Fear Food*. Quoting from chemist Wilbur Atwater's work, entitled *What We Should Eat*, Stacey writes, "In Atwater's system, morality could essentially take the place of enjoyment and taste in the experience of eating; if food were regarded as largely scientific, a fuel for a machine, its spiritual value could be redefined not as the giving of pleasure but the giving of moral fiber."

The school of thought during that time was food served a natural and a spiritual purpose. The natural purpose was to keep people alive. The spiritual purpose was to promote morality through dietary discipline. Our morality is the choices we make and the reasons behind them. Atwater apparently felt a good diet promoted better morals. As Stacey tells it, Atwater was joined in his day by a group of mostly women reformers. She writes:

> At the moment (Atwater) was discoursing on the scientific basis for eating, these women were leading a closely allied movement for scientific cooking, or as it came to be known, "domestic science" (later called home economics). Here too, spiritual considerations ranked high. "The prosperity of a nation depends upon the health and the morals of its citizens, and the health and the morals of a people depend mainly upon the food they eat, and the homes they live in," wrote Ellen H. Richards, one of the founders of the domestic science movement and an instructor in sanitary chemistry at the Massachusetts Institute of Technology, in her 1885 book Food Materials and Their Adulterations. ... The belief that, as one historian puts it, "Good health encouraged a Christian soul and ultimately a moral and strong nation" led one cookbook author of the time to comment, "the system of morals therefore becomes identified with that of cookery."

Stacey notes that those who followed the scientific cookery theory "combined foods based on their nutrients and 'digestibility' rather than their aesthetic appeal." Eating for any reason other than nourishing the body did not factor into their thinking. Stacey's book suggests that these late nineteenth century nutritionists were excited about the future of diet in America. She quotes M.L. Holbrook, author of the 1888 book *Eating For Strength; or Food and Diet in their Relation to Health and Work*:

> "It would almost seem as if the time had nearly arrived when mankind would eat to live, would feed themselves so as to nourish their bodies most perfectly and render themselves capable of the most labor, and least liable to disease. ... There is no doubt but man may double his capacity for work and for enjoyment by improving his dietetic habits." At around this same time, even Mark Twain weighed in on nutrition. He said, "The only way to keep your health is to eat what you don't want, drink what you don't like, and do what you'd rather not."

Fast-forward about a hundred years. That perfect time Holbrook dreamed of never arrived. Instead of eating to nourish our bodies, we too often eat to nurture our wayward emotions. If these insightful scientists and nutritionists were around today, they probably would shake their heads in horror. They might ask, "What happened to all that great information we left behind about food and discipline? Why are people eating the way they do? Don't they know it's killing them? What is that stuff they're eating anyway? It doesn't even look like the real food we ate!" It's easy to see why they would be horrified.

As mankind has "progressed" we have gotten further and further away from the way God intended for us to eat when he put man in a garden and later introduced a little meat into his diet to go with the fruit and vegetables. We have abandoned the spiritual and physical reasons for food and turned it into a fix for heartache. In his book *The Hungry Soul*, author Leon Kass, M.D., refers to the dietary laws in the Bible as God's way of teaching us to control all human appetites. Kass writes, "God sought to protect man from the expansion of his desires beyond the naturally necessary, or from the replacement of desire given by nature with desires given by his own mind and imagination."

Remember, Satan got to Eve by attacking her thought life. He got her to change her mind about what God said. This opened the door to new and false ideas about what she should and should not be eating. Once that was done, he planted disobedience into her mind and her flesh carried out the thought. She did not *need* to eat from the tree of knowledge of good and evil to stay alive. Her motive was not to satisfy natural human hunger. Eve was driven to eat from it for a different reason. She was deceived into thinking it would make her smarter than she already was. Just like so many of us, she was miserable on the other side of that forbidden meal.

We can learn from her mistake. We can see where Eve went wrong. The question is do we know why we miss the mark with our mealtime choices? If we don't know, we'd better find out fast before the chickens behind our emotional eating come home to roost.

Chapter Summary

1. God designed food for fuel, not entertainment.
2. We must fill the emotional needs in our lives with God's Word, not food.
3. God's Word renews our mind and helps us battle contrary thoughts that try to get us to eat toxic foods.

Chapter Seven

Love and War

Question: "On a scale of 1 to 10, describe your energy level at six p.m."
Answer: "Three. I am drained when I come home from work."

Question: "How many cups of coffee do you drink a day?"
Answer: "Usually two to four cups a day. I must have my coffee in the morning. Please don't tell me I have to give up my coffee! I won't be able to function in the morning unless I have my cup of coffee. I *love* coffee and don't think I could live without it."

Question: "How much soda do you drink a day?"
Answer: "At least two to three cans. I don't drink regular soda, though. I *love* diet Coke."

Question: "How many pieces of fruit do you eat each day?"
Answer: Zero to one."

Question: "How many servings of vegetables do you have a day?"
Answer: "Zero. I don't like vegetables and neither do my kids. I have a hard time eating them. You know … although I don't like vegetables, do you want to know what I *love*? I love carbohydrates. I *love* bread and sandwiches. My day would not be complete if I did not have my muffin or bagel with a cup of coffee in the morning."

Question: "Do you eat snacks during the day?"
Answer: "Yes, I have a granola or carb bar for lunch. I usually have a snack after dinner as well."

Question: "What kind of snacks do you have after dinner?"

Answer: "Most of the time, I have ice cream. I just *love* ice cream. It is the one thing I don't think that I could ever give up."

I (Kristy) have had conversations like this with hundreds of clients or prospective clients. This particular client had stopped by the fitness center one Saturday where I worked. She was one of several ladies I spoke to that day. They all told similar stories. But every time I heard the phrase, "I just love ..." my stomach churned and my spirit was burdened. I thought, *Here we are in the midst of a war on health and the casualties of war have fallen in* love *with the enemy.*

Most of us have a favorite food or drink we don't think we can give up. Face it. There are just certain foods that capture our hearts. Whether it is a morning cup of coffee, a mid-day piece of chocolate, or a late night bowl of ice cream, if the thought of living without your comfort food or drink upsets you, you are in a love affair that could end up killing you. Some of the foods you love may hate you. Once they pass your lips and get inside your body, they start working against your organs, cells, and blood supply. They do their damage slowly. Many times people don't catch on until it's too late.

I (Kristy) had a thing for ice cream years ago. It swept me off my feet. I was head over heels in love with it. We had a long affair. In fact, I had a date with a bowl of ice cream every night. Some nights it was a Mr. French Vanilla; other nights it was Mr. Chocolate Chip.

All my friends knew about my affection for ice cream. For my birthday one year, they gave me a gift in honor of my obsession. It was wrapped in lots of paper and I fumbled through it with great anticipation. Finally there it was: a stainless steel, professional ice cream scooper! This gift made my day, as it was not just any old tool for getting my favorite dairy product from the container to the bowl. No. This one was a heavy-duty industrial strength gadget that would not break or bend even when used on ice cream just taken out of the freezer. Wow! How thoughtful! Years later, I realized this present was not so good for me. What I really needed was a gift certificate to a farmer's market.

For years, I (Christine) had a passion for sweets and played the field with pastries. If it was baked with sugar, flour, and lots of fat, I could not resist. Every day I'd cozy up to some kind of dessert. My meal plan was simple:

Breakfast: A doughnut that was already on my desk when I arrived at work — perhaps two if my secretary was feeling particularly benevolent.

Lunch: *Grandma's Cookies* from a vending machine.

Dinner: A blueberry and cream cheese Danish purchased from my favorite bakery on the way home from work.

Thank God I finally got a revelation and went into combat mode. Armed with some literature on the danger of eating this stuff, I got rid of all sugar in my house one day. Even the ketchup and potato chips went in the trash after I read the label and saw they had sugar in them, too.

You're thinking "too radical," right? Well it was not too radical for me. I was a bona fide sugarholic. I was behaving just like someone on drugs or alcohol. I had to have my fix to get me going in the morning and keep me going all day. The only difference between the cocaine addict and me was I could get my drug at the grocery store and they got theirs from a dealer in a back alley. God knew too much of the sweet stuff could be addictive. That's probably why Proverbs 25:27 states, "It is not good to eat much honey."

What food has the key to your heart? What would it take for you to give it up? Does it have to turn on you first? Clog your arteries? Raise your blood sugar level? Drive up your blood pressure? Increase your clothing size by three sizes? Maybe it's not a major idol in your life — just a "little idol." After all, it's only food. It's not like you are bowing down to a pagan god or something. It's just a little chocolate once or twice a day. What's the big deal?

The better question to ask is: Will this "little idol" help you over the long term or hurt you? If Eve had asked this question, maybe paradise would not have been lost. When the serpent tempted her with a little thing like fruit, he was trying to get between Eve and her destiny. He does the same thing today when he tempts us with unhealthy food over and over again. He uses "a little thing" to take over a bigger thing. In Eve's case it was the whole earth. In your case, it could be your whole life and the work God has assigned to you. You might argue, "I don't love food more than I love God." However, you might love it more than you love God's plan for your life.

That's what happened to some of the Hebrews in the wilderness after God brought them out of Egyptian slavery. Their bodies were free but their appetites still felt the pull of Egypt's grocery stores. Shortly after they got a taste of freedom, their first complaint was not having food and drink. This happened right after the praise and worship service recorded in Exodus 15:1-18.

By Exodus 16:3 they were complaining again about food: "Oh, that we had died by the hand of the Lord in the land of Egypt, when we sat by the pots of meat and when we ate bread to the full! For you have brought us out into this wilderness to kill this whole assembly with hunger."

God was patient and met their needs. He rained down bread from heaven and they ate this "manna" for breakfast. At twilight, God covered the camp with quail for their dinner. He instructed Moses to have the people gather the manna "according to each one's need, one omer for each person, according to the number of persons" (Exodus 16:16). "He who gathered much had nothing left over, and he who gathered little had no lack" (Exodus 16:18). Notice the people gathered according to *need*, not appetite.

Fast forward to Numbers 11. By this time, the Jews were *really* missing their favorite foods from Egypt. "Now the mixed multitude who were among them yielded to intense craving; so the children of Israel also wept again and said: 'Who will give us meat to eat? We remember the fish which we ate freely in Egypt, the cucumbers, the melons, the leeks, the onions and the garlic; but now our whole being is dried up; there is nothing at all except this manna before our eyes!' " (Numbers 11:4-6). Notice they were not complaining because they had nothing to eat. God was still sending them manna each day. This crew was upset because they did not have their favorite foods left behind in Egypt.

Historians say the food in ancient Egypt was good. Bread was plentiful. The Nile River was full of fish that was salted, pickled, or split open and sun-dried to prevent spoilage in the warm climate. There were some gourmet dishes, too, such as a recipe for fish marinated in oil and spread with onion, pepper, coriander, and other herbs. Egyptian food was prepared with some of the best spices — rosemary, thyme, sage, dill, mint, marjoram, safflower, mustard seeds, etc.

The fertile Egyptian soil produced a variety of vegetables. Onions, garlic, celery, radishes, lettuce, leeks, parsley, squash, beans, chickpeas, lentils, cucumbers, and peas were used extensively. And those with a sweet tooth were not left wanting. Figs, grapes, melons, raisins, pomegranates, and date palms were among the treats that rounded out the meals.

Fancy pastries existed as well and one Egyptian officer is said to have inscribed the recipe for his favorite cake on the wall of his tomb to assure he would be able to eat it throughout eternity. These are the kinds of meals the Hebrews were probably thinking about when they cried out in Numbers 11. As Bob Brier and Hoyt Hobbs put it in their book, *Daily Life of the Ancient Egyptians*, "Literally thousands of years would pass before anyone would again eat as well and enjoy such variety as the ancient Egyptian."

It was this diet that the Hebrews missed. So the Lord told Moses to answer the people as follows:

***Consecrate yourselves for tomorrow, and you shall eat meat;
for you have wept in the hearing of the Lord, saying, "Who***

will give us meat to eat? For it was well with us in Egypt."
Therefore the Lord will give you meat, and you shall eat.
You shall eat, not one day, nor two days, nor five days, nor
ten days, nor twenty days, but for a whole month, until it
comes out of your nostrils and becomes loathsome to you,
because you have despised the Lord who is among you, and
have wept before Him, saying, "Why did we ever come up
out of Egypt?" Now a wind went out from the Lord, and it
brought quail from the sea and left them fluttering near the
camp ... And the people stayed up all that day, all night, and
all the next day, and gathered the quail (he who gathered
least gathered ten homers); and they spread them out for
themselves all around the camp. But while the meat was still
between their teeth, before it was chewed, the wrath of the
Lord was aroused against the people, and the Lord struck
the people with a very great plague. So he called the name of
that place Kibroth Hattaavah, because there they buried the
people who had yielded to craving.
~ Numbers 11:18-20, 31-34

Those who could not control their appetites died. Spiritually, this was not about the food. It was about the people's inability to trust God to do what was best for them. It was about their inability to think beyond the pleasure of the moment and get a vision for a future in the Promised Land. They loved their desire for meat above their desire for God's best. They trusted their cravings for food over the manna God had chosen for them. It could have been alcohol, drugs, or some other addiction. It just happened to be food.

Ironically, it was the need for food that drove the Hebrews to Egypt in the first place. Remember, there was a famine in the land and Jacob sent his sons there to buy food (Genesis 42:1-3). Over four centuries later (see Exodus 12:40), they were crying about food again. This time it was about "cravings" for what they liked to eat instead of what they needed to stay alive. Perhaps that is why one of the first instructions God gave them involved food, even before they left Egypt:

So you shall observe the Feast of Unleavened Bread, for on
this same day I will have brought your armies out of the

land of Egypt. Therefore you shall observe this day throughout your generations as an everlasting ordinance. In the first month, on the fourteenth day of the month at evening, you shall eat unleavened bread, until the twenty-first day of the month at evening. For seven days no leaven shall be found in your houses, since whoever eats what is leavened, that same person shall be cut off from the congregation of Israel, whether he is a stranger or a native of the land. You shall eat nothing leavened; in all your dwellings you shall eat unleavened bread.
~ Exodus 12:17-20

This restriction has spiritual significance. Giving up something commonly eaten teaches self-control and moderation. It opens a door for something else to take priority — namely, Almighty God. It helps break old habits and creates an opportunity for people to develop new and hopefully better lifestyles.

Having taught numerous nutrition classes to church folk, I (Kristy) have witnessed individuals frantically searching the Scriptures to find just one verse they can use as an excuse to continue eating foods they love even though they know they are not good for their bodies. If you are looking for Bible passages to support your poor dietary habits, then close the book. You won't find it there, for the Bible is the word of life and not death.

In *Secrets of the Vine*, author Bruce Wilkinson uses the parable of the maintenance of a grapevine to explain God's overall purpose for our lives. He explains that every vinedresser plants, prunes, and harvests, in that order, so the grapevine can bear fruit. Like a young grapevine, our purpose in life is to produce fruit for God the vinedresser. "You did not choose Me, but I chose you and appointed you that you should go and bear fruit, and that your fruit should remain, that whatever you ask the Father in My name He may give you" (John 15:16).

If a vine is pruned, it is better able to bring forth fruit. In other words, something closely connected to you is removed during the pruning process so you can be more productive. Imagine that! You might say there is scriptural support for weight loss! As Wilkinson puts it, "God will always prune those things that we slavishly seek first, love most, and begrudge giving up. Again, His goal isn't to plunder or harm, but to liberate us so that we can pursue our true desire — His kingdom. This kind of pruning goes beyond rearranging priorities to the heart of what defines us — the people we love, the possessions we cling to, our deep sense of personal rights. These are the very arenas God must rule if we are to bear fruit." Your diet is just such an arena.

I (Christine) have had to progressively change my mind about what I eat. It has not been easy. God has had to drag me kicking and screaming to the well of nutritional knowledge — and even today I still sometimes drag my feet. Perhaps that is why he opened the door for writing this book. This way the subject is ever before me and hard to ignore, no matter how often I am tempted to overindulge in my favorite foods.

Breaking away from the bondage of foods you love which do not love you may be difficult at first. Just pray and ask God to help you find a new object of affection at mealtime — one that will nurture and preserve your body. Staying committed to dead food is like staying in a physically abusive relationship. You must act wisely. Protect yourself. Don't let the food you love eat your life away. Love it occasionally if you must and from afar but do not take this serpent to your bosom. It will eventually bite you. The children of Israel learned this the hard way. Their bodies were out of Egypt but their minds were still there. They were committed to a way of eating that had strings attached. Those "strings" were the chains of slavery. They ate well in Egypt but boy, did they pay a high price! Thank God for coming to the rescue!

He saved them from Pharaoh and took them through a wilderness boot camp to prepare them for battle in the Promised Land. But they had to give up some old thoughts and some old ways of eating. God had a plan to develop them in spirit, soul, and body. That is why he gave them laws dealing with their relationship with him, their relationship with others, and their relationship with their flesh. Most of the laws dealing with the flesh placed a heavy emphasis on food — what to eat and not eat. In fact, all the laws involved some kind of sacrifice.

The people sacrificed animals to atone for their sins before God (see Leviticus 1). They sacrificed property to right a wrong committed against another person (see Leviticus 6). And they sacrificed food to discipline their flesh and stay healthy in the wilderness (see Leviticus 11). God knew food could be a stronghold in their lives. A stronghold is a place dominated by a particular habit, belief, or characteristic. If you have one contrary to how God wants you to live, ask him to help you tear it down no matter how innocent or harmless it may seem on the surface. In the kingdom of God when you give up something not good for you, you open the door to receive God's best.

I (Kristy) meet with people frequently who have food strongholds and don't know it. It's my job to work hard to help people tear them down. One day during the "but I just love ..." part of a nutrition consultation with a client, the client screamed, "You're killing me!" when I told her she had to stop drinking diet soda and eating fast food in order to lose weight and regain her health. I responded, "No, I am saving your life!"

Chapter Summary

1. The food you love may not love you.
2. God is not pleased when we put our cravings above his best for us.
3. Giving up a food you "love" is a sacrificial investment in your future.

Chapter Eight

Feast or Fast?

'Twas the night before Christmas when all through the house,
Not a creature was stirring, not even a mouse.
The children were nestled all snug in their beds, while visions of sugar
plums danced through their heads.
~ Excerpt from poem, *The Night Before Christmas* by Clement Clarke
Moore

Most holidays are nothing more than opportunities for gluttony. What do gingerbread houses and green bean casseroles have to do with an occasion Webster defines as a "Holy Day; a day marked by a general suspension of work in commemoration of an event"? The Bible refers to holidays as "feasts" but not the kind where food is the object of affection. At feasts, God is glorified instead of our stomachs. Food had no role or only a symbolic role in the annual feasts designated by God. But these days we eat our way through the calendar every year.

New Year's Day: For dinner, it's black-eyed peas for "good luck." Southern recipes for black-eyed peas call for ham hocks or pieces of fat back to add "flavor." Other items on the menu may include a couple of meat entrees, potato salad, macaroni and cheese, cakes, and pies. To get through the football games, it's chips and multiple dips, chili, popcorn, nachos, quesadillas, cookies, beer, punch, sodas, etc.

Super Bowl Sunday: Not officially a holiday, but because it's another occasion to overeat, it feels like a holiday. The menu is typical football game fare – pizza, sodas, chips, etc.

President's Day: There are no special foods associated with this holiday. Many people just shop 'til they drop and then pig out at the mall or at their favorite restaurant to celebrate all the bargains they got. The closest they come to remembering a deceased president on this day is when they hand over cash for their purchases.

Valentine's Day: Oh, that wonderful day set aside to express love! How do we do it? We buy tons and tons of chocolate candy and urge people we say we care about to eat as much of it as possible.

Fat Tuesday (40 days prior to Easter): This day is officially dedicated to excess (food, promiscuity, whatever). It is the day before the beginning of Lent, the forty days preceding the commemoration of Christ's crucifixion and resurrection. Many people "give up" something for Lent like chocolate or meat. This act of sacrifice is biblically sound and can be very spiritually rewarding. It won't be, however, if we treat the sacrifice as if we're doing God a favor, feel all holy about it, count the days until it's over and then go back to the same unhealthy lifestyles we had before Lent.

Easter: Many Christians celebrate the resurrection of Christ on this day. Some people dress up in new clothes, go to church services, and rush from the sanctuary to the nearest restaurant or a home-cooked meal. Ham, hot cross buns, pineapple upside-down cake, over-cooked vegetables, and starchy side dishes are among the traditional foods served on this occasion.

The secular component of Easter is Satan's little counterfeit. Its traditions (bunnies and eggs) are derived from ancient worship of the Babylonian fertility goddess Ishtar. Since bunnies and eggs are not very tempting as dietary weapons of destruction, the candy industry saves the day for Satan by providing several sweets for kids to eat to their hearts' content. They're presented very nicely, too, in beautifully decorated buckets and baskets. It's just another season for business to get a boost, our teeth to take a beating, and our bodies to pick up a few more pounds.

Mothers Day: It's a time to honor mom. She's showered with flowers, jewelry, mushy greeting cards, and, of course, the obligatory meal. Perhaps it is brunch at a fancy restaurant. Or it may be a home-cooked dinner courtesy of the honoree. Once again, food is a key component.

Memorial Day: At this time, American people are supposed to honor the country's war dead. Instead, Memorial Day has deteriorated into another food fest signaling the start of summer with tons of barbecue, starchy side dishes, sugary drinks, alcohol, and multiple desserts.

Independence Day (July 4th): What a wonderful occasion — the day thirteen British colonies in North America declared their independence and became the United States of America. We commemorate this historic moment with still more food and drink (hot dogs, sweets, more barbecue, sodas, beer, etc.).

The city of Chicago goes all out for July 4th. Each year, it hosts the ever popular "Taste of Chicago." Several local restaurants openly market their best cuisine at a huge outdoor picnic in the park that lasts about two weeks. Guests buy tickets and use them to purchase samples of any food that catches their eye.

Instead of waving red, white, and blue flags at this event, many Chicagoans wave giant turkey legs and empty beer glasses. The hot topics of discussion at "The Taste," as it is lovingly called, are not democracy's fate or the state of the nation but which vendor has the best rib tips and how to avoid waiting in the long lines to taste them. From pizza to pork, whatever saturated fat your arteries desire can be found at the "Taste of Chicago." This event alone, no doubt, helped place Chicago in the number two spot on the nation's fattest cities list published in 2003 by *Men's Fitness* magazine. That year, Houston was number one for the third time in a row.

Labor Day: This is the day set aside for Americans to celebrate the country's workforce and organized labor's role in improving job conditions. For the most part, we treat it as an occasion for one more barbecue before the weather turns cold.

Halloween: This is the "Festival of the Dead," when children and adults dress up in costumes (the scarier the better) and knock on doors to collect candy. Children consider the holiday a success if they collect enough sweets to keep them high on sugar for several weeks. In 2004, Americans spent two billion dollars on Halloween candy. The holiday has some dark paganistic origins but it has been repackaged for marketing and other unholy purposes as just "a day for fun" — a time for people to let their hair down and be a little crazy. In terms of spending, it is the second biggest holiday after Christmas. H. Daniel Wilson's book, *Why the Saved Don't Celebrate Halloween*, notes:

> (Halloween) was started in Europe by the ancient people called the Celts and their priests who were known as the Druids. Halloween was a pagan holiday in which the transition from light of summer to the darkness of winter was celebrated. It was also a time of prayer and sacrifice to the false god Samana (the lord of death) also known as the grim reaper. On this night, tradition says the spirits of the dead rose, and along with them, for this one night only, other creatures also came out (witches, ghouls, demons). Tradition says on this night, so the spirits would not destroy their crop or kill their cattle, people had decided to give their ghouls a treat (or

food) so the ghoul would not give them a trick and destroy their goods. This is how the term "Trick or Treat" was established.

The history of Halloween also includes reports of child sacrifices to Satan. Many people do not believe this goes on. Nevertheless, Satan's mission to steal, kill, and destroy gets a big boost on October 31 in more subtle ways. He uses sacks of candy loaded with sugar and artificial colors to strike a blow against good health. We see the fruits of his labor in the rising number of children challenged with obesity and diabetes.

Thanksgiving: This holiday has the potential to put God first. After all, it is the official day to give thanks for all of our blessings in the good old USA. Unfortunately, it has changed from a day of thanksgiving to "Turkey Day" — a time to pay respect to a big bird soaked in butter and stuffed with bread. "Bless the Lord, O my soul, and forget not all His benefits" (Psalm 103:2) seems to have taken a back seat to "Pass the gravy and cranberry sauce."

Christmas: The time formally designated to celebrate Jesus Christ's birthday has deteriorated into just about anything but. Many activities during this season have nothing to do with the world-changing events in that Bethlehem stable 2,000 years ago. Food bondage takes hold in earnest this time of year, so much so that the majority of New Year's resolutions involve commitments to lose weight after all the overeating that goes on between Thanksgiving and Christmas.

The season is not only known for overeating but also for increased commercialism, excessive spending, and legal battles over nativity scenes on government property, Christmas carols in public schools, and whether "Merry Christmas" should be replaced with the more benign "Happy Holidays" so as not to offend people of other religions. But despite the culture wars, most folks somehow manage to get past these differences and help eat the Christmas goodies. People of all faiths and no faith bond around the buffet table and give a bow to the god of greed.

In ancient Israel, holidays were celebrated quite differently. First of all, they never were on the same date because they followed the lunar calendar on which special dates occur depending on the phases of the moon. These "feast days" involved restraint, not indulgence. Instead of making eating the centerpiece, they were designed by God to teach each new generation about who he is, remind Israel of its role in the Messianic prophecies, and keep them set apart as a holy nation, as God's chosen people. Self-gratification played no part in the feast traditions.

The feasts of the Lord are detailed in Leviticus 23 (see also references in Exodus 23:14-16 and Deuteronomy 16:1-15). The Lord began by telling Moses how the people were to observe the Sabbath. They were to work six days and rest on the seventh (Leviticus 23:1-3). No food is mentioned. God then told Moses how to observe seven feasts saying, "These are the feasts of the Lord, holy convocations which you shall proclaim at their appointed times" (Leviticus 23:4).

The Feast of Passover

On the fourteenth day of the first month at twilight is the Lord's Passover. ~ Leviticus 23:5

This holy day commemorates how God saved Israel when the last of ten plagues against Egypt killed that nation's first born but passed over the Hebrews. It was the final blow that forced Pharaoh to let the Israelites go. Before the death angel swept through the land, God told Moses to have the Hebrews take a lamb "without blemish, a male of the first year" (Exodus 12:5), kill it in the evening, put its blood over the door and on the side posts, roast it and eat the lamb with unleavened bread and bitter herbs.

The meal was symbolic of deliverance (the blood of the lamb), victory over sin (unleavened bread), and the harshness of slavery (bitter herbs). It also was practical as the Jews needed physical strength for their journey out of Egypt. Jesus kept the Passover during the meal Christians call the "Last Supper" (Matthew 26:17-29). Occasionally the feast, which always falls on the first full moon of the spring, coincides with Easter Sunday.

Feast of Unleavened Bread

And on the fifteenth day of the same month is the Feast of Unleavened Bread to the Lord; seven days you must eat unleavened bread. ~ Leviticus 23:6

The seven-day Feast of Unleavened Bread begins on the day after Passover. The first day is a holy convocation, in which no work was to be done. Burnt offerings to the Lord were made for seven days, followed by a final day of holy convocation on the seventh day. During this entire period, unleavened bread was eaten. Leaven represented sin and evil. This was a time to focus on holiness.

On the practical side, the unleavened bread represented the haste with which the Jews left Egypt. There was simply no time to let the bread rise. Its taste was irrelevant. Again, God had a prophetic point to make. It was fulfilled in Jesus, whose body was broken to redeem the world. This act was symbolic of a time when human life would not be sustained by bread alone, but by Jesus, who is the "Bread of Life."

The Feast of Firstfruits

Speak to the children of Israel, and say to them, "When you come into the land which I give to you and reap its harvest, then you shall bring a sheaf of the firstfruits of your harvest to the priest. He shall wave the sheaf before the Lord, to be accepted on your behalf; on the day after the Sabbath the priest shall wave it." ~ Leviticus 23:10-11

Through this offering, God wanted the Israelites to acknowledge the fertility of the land he had given them. In addition to a field offering, a young lamb without blemish was to be given as a burnt offering. Grain mixed with oil and a drink offering of wine was also to be given. The people were not allowed to eat grains or bread until the burnt offerings were made (see Leviticus 23:14). Firstfruits represented the resurrection of Christ and the future resurrection of the entire church. Prophetic symbolism and abstinence were the hallmarks of this holy day.

The Feast of Harvest or Pentecost

And you shall count for yourselves from the day after the Sabbath, from the day that you brought the sheaf of the wave offering; seven Sabbaths shall be completed. Count fifty days to the day after the seventh Sabbath; then you shall offer a new grain offering to the Lord. ~ Leviticus 23:15-16

The Lord required the following offerings for this feast: two wave loaves baked with leaven; as a burnt offering, seven lambs without blemish of the first year, one young bullock, and two rams; a meat offering; drink offerings; one kid of goats as a sin offering;

and two lambs of the first year as a peace offering. Finally, the Lord said, "When you reap the harvest of your land, you shall not wholly reap the corners of your field when you reap, nor shall you gather any gleaning from your harvest. You shall leave them for the poor and for the stranger" (Leviticus 23:22). In sum, this holy day was about giving to the Lord and to others in need, and forecasting future events that would shake the world such as salvation of sinful man — both Jews and Gentiles (the two loaves) — and the New Testament Pentecost when the Holy Spirit would be poured out.

Feast of Trumpets — Rosh Hashanah

Speak to the children of Israel, saying, "In the seventh month, on the first day of the month, you shall have a sabbath-rest, a memorial of blowing of trumpets, a holy convocation. ~ Leviticus 23:24

The trumpet or ram's horn was used to call field workers immediately to worship. It was a time of rest. An offering by fire was made to the Lord. Another foreshadow of things to come was recorded in 1 Corinthians 15:52: "In a moment, in the twinkling of an eye, at the last trumpet. For the trumpet will sound, and the dead will be raised incorruptible, and we shall be changed."

Day of Atonement — Yom Kippur

Also the tenth day of this seventh month shall be the Day of Atonement. It shall be a holy convocation for you; you shall afflict your souls, and offer an offering made by fire to the Lord. ~ Leviticus 23:27

The Day of Atonement is the holiest of all the Jewish feast days. On this solemn occasion, the high priest would enter the Holy of Holies, where God dwelt. He was the only one who could enter this part of the tabernacle and was responsible for sprinkling blood on the mercy seat of the Ark of the Covenant as atonement for Israel's sins (Leviticus 16:2-34). This was such a serious event that, according to tradition, a rope was tied around the high priest's ankle so that if the sacrifice was not acceptable to God and the priest was struck dead, he could be pulled from the Holy of Holies. Jews were not allowed to work on this day. Those who did any work, such as lifting something too heavy, were cut off. This solemn occasion is representative of our spiritual cleansing through the precious blood of Jesus.

The Feast of Tabernacles

Speak to the children of Israel, saying: "The fifteenth day of this seventh month shall be the Feast of Tabernacles for seven days to the Lord. You shall dwell in booths for seven days. All who are native Israelites shall dwell in booths, that your generations may know that I made the children of Israel dwell in booths, when I brought them out of the land of Egypt. ~ *Leviticus 23:34, 42-43*

The first and last days of this feast were set aside for rest. In between, various sacrifices and offerings were made and the people rejoiced before the Lord for seven days (Leviticus 23:40). God said he ordered this feast so new generations would know how the Israelites had to live in tents or "booths" in the wilderness after he brought them out of Egypt.

All rituals associated with the Jewish feasts had one thing many of our holiday observations lack: divine focus. Sacrifice. Rest. Remembrance. Prophetic forecasting. Atonement and rejoicing before the Lord, versus eating too much, drinking too much, and spending too much. They gave to the Lord as opposed to giving to themselves. They kept their eyes on the Lord and the future.

What is your focus during our holidays, especially those with religious significance? All holidays — even the secular celebrations — are opportunities to serve God and serve as an example of his presence in the earth. In the United States, Americans have overshadowed the true significance of major holidays underneath a variety of different foods. Why is it when it comes to a major holiday on which we are to celebrate a great day in history, the focus is solely on what is going to be eaten? Our holidays, which were designated to commemorate historical events, are taken far out of context. Don't let the holidays become just another occasion to eat. Instead of fixing your eyes on the Virginia ham and pumpkin pie, fix your heart on the Lord who makes the occasion and the meal possible.

It is time to take a fresh approach to holiday celebrations. Instead of feasting on everything in sight, decide to make it a day of fasting. Perhaps you could fast your favorite food on this day or make it a fast covering multiple days. Whatever you do, make the Word of God your main course and represent him in all you do during these special times.

Chapter Summary

1. Major holidays are nothing more than big food orgies for many people.

2. These special times were set aside to celebrate important milestones in human history and most of them were born out of religious or spiritual convictions, which is why they are called "holidays" from the root word *holy*.

3. If we were to follow the biblical "holy-day" traditions, we would acknowledge the time with fasting and praying versus eating and partying.

Kristy Dotson & Christine Tennon

Chapter Nine

Denying Yourself

"Tomorrow, this church is beginning a twenty-one-day fast."

When my pastor made that announcement from the pulpit one Sunday morning, I (Christine) was frightened. Of course, participation was voluntary. There was absolutely no pressure to join in except the religious pressure I brought on myself.

I thought, *How could I possibly go without food even for a day, let alone twenty-one days! Surely I will die!*

Then the pastor said, "It's a Daniel fast (see Daniel 10:2-3). No meat or sweets."

I thought, *Oh, I could handle that. But I can't give up my daily banana nut muffin. Is that a sweet? No. It's probably better classified as bread and fruit. Besides, it's made with dark flour. It's healthy. So I should be okay. But maybe I should call my doctor to see if he thinks fasting is unhealthy for me. And what about treats? Since I'm giving up sweets, I've got to have some kind of treat! I also work hard. There is no way I can keep my energy up without something sweet. What if I pass out at work from low blood sugar or something?*

The Bible says you're supposed to fast in secret. If I pass out at work, I'll have to tell them why and that would be a sin, wouldn't it? Maybe I should only fast when I'm not at work. Otherwise, if my co-workers find out, they'll think I'm crazy. God understands the challenges of modern living. He made food for my pleasure. It was easier to fast back in Bible days. They did not have much to eat anyway. They were used to going without food.

Instead of food, maybe I'll just fast television for twenty-one days — at least the news. I've got to see Law & Order *and Christian TV. That's it! I'll do a Daniel fast when I'm not at work and then I'll skip everything on television except my favorite shows. That should work. Whew! I'm glad there is freedom in Christ.*

But I wasn't free. I was in bondage to my eating lifestyle. The thought of giving up certain foods — especially those I liked — for twenty-one days was simply unacceptable. It never occurred to me that designing a fast that allowed me to keep my creature comforts was not really a fast. It was nothing more than a religious exercise — a slight change in my daily routine that would give me bragging rights with the rest of the church folks. It meant I did not understand the power of fasting. But most importantly, it meant I was not desperate — not like some of the folks in the Bible who would skip a few meals and go down in sackcloth and ashes in a heartbeat when their backs were against the wall. They used fasting as a spiritual weapon — just like God intended.

Combating Rebellion: Faced with thousands of unruly ex-slaves and a wilderness journey, Moses fasted forty days and forty nights when he went up to Mt. Sinai to receive the law and commandments from God (Exodus 24:18; Deuteronomy 9:9). When he came down from the mountain and saw the Israelites had made an idol to worship, he fasted another forty days and forty nights because he was afraid God would destroy the people. He also prayed. And as Moses put it, the Lord "listened" to him and let the people live (Deuteronomy 9:18-19).

When the prophet Jonah warned the people of Nineveh they would be overthrown in forty days because of their wickedness, they repented and proclaimed a fast (Jonah 3:4-5). God relented and did not destroy them. (Jonah 3:10)

Combating Sin: Fasting was part of the Jewish law and was instrumental in the act of repentance. Leviticus 16:29-30 says: "This shall be a statute forever for you: In the seventh month, on the tenth day of the month, you shall afflict your souls, and do not work at all, whether a native of your own country or a stranger who dwells among you. For on that day the priest shall make atonement for you, to cleanse you, that you may be clean from all your sins before the Lord."

Combating Defeat: Nehemiah, a Jewish patriot, during the time of Israel's enslavement by Persian King Artaxerxes, became so distressed and frustrated when he heard the wall of Jerusalem had been broken down that he fasted and prayed. At the time, Nehemiah was serving as the king's cupbearer. He asked God for mercy when he went before his master. A few months later, the king not only gave Nehemiah permission to go to Jerusalem and rebuild the wall, he also gave him access to resources needed for the project! (Nehemiah 1:1-11, 2:1-9) Chalk up another victory as a result of fasting and praying!

Combating Loss: King David fasted when the son he had with Bathsheba was sick. Bathsheba had been married to Uriah, one of David's soldiers. When David started an affair with her and Bathsheba became pregnant, he arranged for Uriah to be killed in battle (2 Samuel 11:15). The prophet Nathan told David that as a result of this sin, the "sword" would never depart from his house and the child he and Bathsheba conceived would surely die. The child did die despite David's fast.

Some of you might not be encouraged by this story. After all, David gave up food and still did not get what he wanted. What's the point of this bit of biblical history? The point is to help us better understand the purpose of fasting and when it is effective.

When people in the Bible fasted, they were typically seeking God's help with a serious problem that was not their fault. But David's problem was a consequence of his sin. His son got sick because David committed murder and adultery. These sins opened the door to judgment. Repentance is the remedy for judgment. Repentance removes the stain of sin that separates us from a Holy God. Repentance moves God's heart to forgiveness. Fasting moves his hand to deliverance and blessing.

David was using fasting at a time when repentance seemed to be more in order. And although fasting did not alter the judgment resulting from David's sin, it did apparently open the door to a blessing. David and Bathsheba had another son. This child, Solomon, was loved of God and blessed with wisdom and riches (2 Samuel 12:1-24). Indeed, David's fast was not a waste of time.

Combating Grief: When King Saul took his life after being wounded in a battle with the Philistines, his attackers fastened his body to a wall for all to see (1 Samuel 31:1-13). David and the men who buried Saul fasted to mourn Saul's death (2 Samuel 1:1-12).

Combating Enemies: When King Jehoshaphat got word one day that "a great multitude" of Syrian soldiers was coming to do battle with him, he "proclaimed a fast throughout all Judah" (2 Chronicles 20:2-3). He also gathered the people and prayed. Then the Spirit of the Lord came upon one of the Jewish priests, who declared, "Do not be afraid nor dismayed because of this great multitude, for the battle is not yours, but God's" (2 Chronicles 20:15).

On the day of battle, Jehoshaphat appointed those who would sing to the Lord and those who would praise him. When the people began to sing and praise, the Lord confused Judah's enemies and they fought against each other until every one of them was dead. Jehoshaphat defeated his enemies with fasting, praise, and worship instead of natural weapons. He and his people then spent three days collecting the spoils of war, including precious jewelry and other valuables (2 Chronicles 20:20-25).

Several things happened during this event. There was corporate prayer, a Word from God spoken by the priest, worship, praise, and ultimately victory without even having to fight. But first, there was fasting. You have to wonder what would have happened if they had started with corporate prayer and skipped the fast.

Jews enslaved by King Artaxerxes fasted for protection on their journey to Jerusalem to beautify the house of the Lord (Ezra 8:21-23, 31; 7:11-28). Ezra, a priest who led the group, describes how they went about it.

> *Then I proclaimed a fast there at the river of Ahava, that we might humble ourselves before our God, to seek from Him the right way for us and our little ones and all our possessions. For I was ashamed to request of the king an escort of soldiers and horsemen to help us against the enemy on the road, because we had spoken to the king, saying, "The hand of our God is upon all those for good who seek Him, but his power and His wrath are against all those who forsake Him." So we fasted and entreated our God for this, and He answered our prayer. ... Then we departed from the river of Ahava on the twelfth day of the first month, to go to Jerusalem. And the hand of our God was upon us, and He delivered us from the hand of the enemy and from ambush along the road. ~ Ezra 8:21-23, 31*

This group was determined to fulfill God's divine purpose and they used fasting to get to Jerusalem and work on rebuilding the Lord's temple. Mission accomplished, minus a few meals.

Combating Evil: Esther's fast was a matter of life and death. She was made queen in the court of Ahasuerus, king of the Medo-Persian Empire. But he did not know she was a Jew. Haman, one of the king's princes, became upset because Esther's Uncle Mordecai, a devout Jew, would not bow down to him. So Haman got the king to order the murder of all Jews.

"And in every province where the king's command and decree arrived, there was great mourning among the Jews, with fasting, weeping, and wailing; and many lay in sackcloth and ashes" (Esther 4:3). When Esther learned what was going on, she sent Mordecai the following message:

> *"Go, gather all the Jews who are present in Shushan, and fast for me; neither eat nor drink for three days, night or day. My maids and I will fast likewise. And so I will go to the*

king which is against the law; and if I perish, I perish!" So Mordecai went his way and did according to all that Esther commanded him. ~ Esther 4:16-17

Esther literally had her neck on the line. Jewish historian Josephus writes in *The Antiquities of the Jews 11/6*: "The king had made a law, that none of his own people should approach him unless they were called, when he sat upon his throne; and men with axes in their hands, stood round about his throne, in order to punish such as approached to him without being called. However, the king sat with a golden scepter in his hand, which he held out when he had a mind to save anyone of those that approached to him without being called; and he who touched it was free from danger." When Esther approached the king without being summoned, God granted her favor with the king who extended the scepter when she drew near to him.

In the end, Haman was hanged on the very gallows he had prepared for Mordecai, the king revoked the murder decree, and Mordecai assumed a position of great honor in the king's court. This combination of faith and fasting saved God's chosen people from being killed and protected the lineage through which Christ would come nearly five hundred years later.

Combating Corruption: Daniel fasted and prayed to stay true to the Jewish law while a captive in Babylon under King Nebuchadnezzar. Daniel was one of the Hebrew princes forced to serve in the palace.

And the king appointed for them a daily provision of the king's delicacies and of the wine which he drank and three years of training for them, so that at the end of that time they might serve before the king. ... But Daniel purposed in his heart that he would not defile himself with the portion of the king's delicacies, nor with the wine, which he drank; therefore he requested of the chief of the eunuchs that he might not defile himself. ~Daniel 1:5, 8

The chief was afraid the king would chop off the chief's head if Daniel and his three Hebrew friends ended up looking worse than the other men who ate the king's food. But Daniel understood the health benefits of fasting and said, "Please test your servants for ten days, and let them give us vegetables to eat and water to drink. Then let our appearance be examined before you, and the appearance of the young men who eat the portion of the king's delicacies; and as you see fit, so deal with your servants" (Daniel 1:12-13). The chief gave in. And after ten days, Daniel and his friends looked "better and fatter in flesh" than all the young men who ate the king's food. God also blessed them with wisdom, literary skill, and knowledge, and gave Daniel the understanding of dreams and visions (Daniel 1:14-17).

If ever there were an excuse to pig out, being a slave is one of them. But Daniel had a vision for a better life and preserved himself so he could enjoy it when it came. Josephus writes Daniel and his Jewish friends "had their souls in some measure more pure, and less burdened, and so fitter for learning and had their bodies in better trim for hard labor" by avoiding the food from the king's table (*The Antiquities of the Jews 10/10*). Fasting played a major role in Daniel's lifestyle throughout his captivity.

Combating Lack of Knowledge: Daniel fasted and prayed after reading Jeremiah's prophesies that Israel was to remain enslaved by other nations for seventy years (Daniel 9:3). At the end of that fast, the angel Gabriel showed up to help Daniel understand the end-time prophecy of the "seventy weeks" leading up to the return of Christ (Daniel 9). Gabriel told Daniel, "At the beginning of your supplications the command went out, and I have come to tell you, for you are greatly beloved; therefore consider the matter, and understand the vision" (Daniel 9:23).

Again, look at what skipping a few meals, praying, and earnestly seeking God's wisdom can do. Perhaps the same thing would have happened if Daniel had continued eating while praying. Only God knows. But Daniel got the information he was seeking after praying *and* fasting.

Combating Distress: Daniel 10 records what is probably Daniel's most famous fast. It was the third year of the reign of Cyrus, King of Persia. Daniel was sorrowful because of a vision he had had but did not understand.

In those days I, Daniel, was mourning three full weeks. I ate no pleasant food, no meat or wine came into my mouth, nor did I anoint myself at all, till three whole weeks were fulfilled. Now on the twenty-fourth day of the first month, as I was by the side of the great river, that is, the Tigris, I lifted my eyes and looked, and behold a certain man clothed in linen whose waist was girded with gold of Uphaz! His body was like beryl, his face like the appearance of lightning, his eyes like torches of fire, his arms and feet like burnished bronze in color, and the sound of the his words like the voice of a multitude. ~ *Daniel 10:2-6*

And he said to me, "O Daniel, man greatly beloved, understand the words that I speak to you, and stand upright, for I have now been sent to you." While he was speaking this word to me, I stood trembling. Then he said to me, "Do not fear Daniel, for from the first day that you set your heart to understand, and to humble yourself before your God, your words were heard; and I have come because of your words. But the prince of the kingdom of Persia withstood me twenty-one days; and behold, Michael, one of the chief princes, came to help me, for I had been left alone there with the kings of Persia. Now I have come to make you understand what will happen to your people in the latter days, for the vision refers to many days yet to come."
~ *Daniel 10:11-14*

There are some powerful lessons in this passage. First, the same angel Gabriel who responded to Daniel in Daniel 9, heard Daniel's petition on the FIRST day of this fast! Truly the angels wait on us to speak God's Word (see Psalm 103:20). Second, nothing had changed in Daniel's world at the end of the twenty-one days. But there was a whole lot going on in the unseen world!

God's angels were battling it out with "the prince of the kingdom of Persia." This prince refers to the ruling demonic spirit over that part of the world. Remember, Daniel was living under an earthly Persian king at that time so he would have known if Gabriel had been referring to a fight with this human king. Clearly this was not a battle visible to the human eyes. Third, Daniel got divine direction from his heavenly visitor about events still to come.

Daniel's fast set angels into immediate action. It led to a battle in the heavens between God's angels and the forces of darkness, and ultimately led to the delivery of information from God about end-time events. All of this because Daniel mixed faith with flesh control. It is a good thing he was more interested in the things of God during this time than he was in food.

Combating Culture: After Jesus was born, Mary and Joseph brought him to Jerusalem to present him to the Lord and offer a sacrifice according to the Law of Moses (Luke 2:22-24). In the temple was Anna, a prophetess, who "did not depart from the temple, but served God with fastings and prayers night and day … gave thanks to the Lord, and spoke of Him to all those who looked for redemption in Jerusalem" (Luke 2:37-38). This was obviously a woman who was tired of life in Jerusalem as she knew it, and prayed to God for a new day. The followers of John the Baptist were also at odds with the culture during this time and set themselves apart by calling on people to repent. In Matthew 9:14, they told Jesus they fasted "often."

Combating Unbelief: A man with an epileptic son came to Jesus one day and said:

"So I brought him to your disciples, but they could not cure him." Then Jesus answered and said, "O faithless and perverse generation, how long shall I be with you? How long shall I bear with you? Bring him here to me." And Jesus rebuked the demon, and it came out of him; and the child was cured from that very hour. Then the disciples came to Jesus privately and said, "Why could we not cast it out?" So Jesus said to them, "Because of your unbelief; for assuredly, I say to you, if you have faith as a mustard seed, you will say to this mountain, 'Move from here to there,' and it will move; and nothing will be impossible for you. However this kind does not go out except by prayer and fasting." ~ Matthew 17:16-21

Prayer, faith *and* fasting were necessary to win this battle with this demon. Prayer without fasting could not get the job done and fasting without prayer couldn't either. But the two together built faith and faith is the vehicle that brings about God's will on earth.

Combating Distraction: The first recorded attack against the adult Jesus was food-related. Jesus fasted before he launched his ministry. Satan tried the same trick on him that he used on Eve in the Garden of Eden.

Then Jesus was led up by the Spirit into the wilderness to be tempted by the devil. And when he had fasted forty days and

forty nights, afterward he was hungry. Now when the tempter came to Him, he said, "If you are the Son of God, command that these stones become bread." But he answered and said, "It is written, 'Man shall not live by bread alone, but by every word that proceeds from the mouth of God.'"
~ Matthew 4:1-4

The Apostle Paul, after his conversion to Christianity on the Damascus road, did not eat or drink for three days. Neither could he see. Later, the disciple Ananias laid hands on Paul, known then as Saul, and Paul's sight was restored. Without his sight and without food to distract him, he no doubt was able to hear from God during those three days (Acts 9:1-18). After Saul spent some time with the disciples, he immediately preached in the synagogues that Christ is the Son of God (Acts 9:19-20). This was quite a transformation for a man who had been a passionate enemy of the church.

Combating the Status Quo: In Acts 10:30-32, Cornelius a devout Roman centurion was fasting. He was not even Jewish but he kept their traditions and was obviously seeking to change his life. Cornelius shared his story this way: "Four days ago I was fasting until this hour; and at the ninth hour I prayed in my house and behold, a man stood before me in bright clothing and said, 'Cornelius, your prayer has been heard, and your alms are remembered in the sight of God. Send therefore to Joppa and call Simon here, whose surname is Peter. He is lodging in the house of Simon, a tanner, by the sea. When he comes he will speak to you.'"

Here was an unsaved man seeking to change his life. He knew enough from observing the Jews that their God could get things done. When Peter showed up at Cornelius's house and preached the gospel, Cornelius and his whole household were saved (Acts 10:44-48).

Fasting opens the door to the supernatural. That's no doubt the reason the Apostle Paul was able to spread the gospel so effectively. He fasted often (2 Corinthians 6:5; 11:27).

Combating Uncertainty: Certain teachers and prophets at Antioch fasted while ministering to the Lord. During that time they received direction by the Holy Spirit to send Barnabas and Saul out to do the work God had assigned them to do (Acts 13:1-3).

Combating Opposition to the Gospel: Paul and Barnabas fasted, prayed, and appointed church elders after withstanding attacks while preaching the gospel in Iconium and Lystra (Acts 14:1-23).

Again and again we see how fasting invoked the power of God — power that opened doors, calmed fears, defeated enemies, changed hearts, provided protection, and helped spread the gospel to the world. I wish I'd known this when my pastor called that Daniel fast years ago. It probably would not have turned out to be an exercise in futility.

What heavenly revelations are we missing because we do not fast or because we fast and do not understand fasting? What mountains are we failing to move? What spiritual battles are being lost because we do not take authority over our flesh? Miraculously I (Christine) did learn something from my little compromise fast. I learned God's hand did not move when I fasted for the wrong reason (see Isaiah 58:3-9; Zechariah 7:1-7, 13). I also learned fasting is not about changing God's way of doing things. It is about changing my understanding of who God is, how he moves, and how I need to change in order to align my life with God's will.

Why fasting? Because it humbles us. Humility makes our voice heard on high by God (Ezra 8:21). It is a way of showing God by our actions that we do not trust our own strength to get us through troubled times, but we trust in him. In Psalm 69:10, David talks about chastening his soul with fasting. When we chasten our souls, we discipline our thoughts and emotions. When our thoughts are under control, we can make better decisions about life.

Ultimately, fasting is about change. Christians are often encouraged to pray for change but rarely are we told to fast for change. Fasting not only changes our minds but our bodies. It causes weight loss, cleanses the digestive track, helps remove harmful toxins and waste, increases energy levels, makes cravings for unhealthy food (especially sugar) go away, and increases mental clarity.

If going without food for a while can get us to a better spiritual and physical place, then fasting is well worth it. In the beginning, a lack of self-control with food plunged the world into chaos. Since eating forbidden food robbed us of life in paradise, it stands to reason that passing up food for an appointed time should be a key weapon in the fight to reclaim all our privileges as God's children. Decide today to make fasting a part of your spiritual and physical battle plan to gain and maintain good health.

Chapter Summary

1. Fasting is a powerful weapon in spiritual warfare.
2. Giving up food or certain foods for periods of time can help us overcome many common problems such as confusion, distress, grief, evil, unbelief, enemies, health problems, etc.
3. Fasting changes us and moves the hand of God on our behalf.

Chapter Ten

Lessons from the Tabernacle

And I heard a loud voice from heaven saying, "Behold, the tabernacle of God is with men, and He will dwell with them, and they shall be His people. God Himself will be with them and be their God." ~ Revelation 21:3

God is everywhere. But after Adam and Eve sinned, communicating with mankind face-to-face without barriers ended. So God had to come up with another way to personally interact with people. He did this by designating three locations on earth as special dwelling places for him:

1. The tabernacle
2. The temple
3. Inside those who have received Jesus Christ as Lord and Savior (Romans 8:9-11, 1 Corinthians 3:16)

The tabernacle was basically a tent with three sections that God told Moses to build in the wilderness as a place of worship after the Jews left Egypt. Years later, it was replaced with the temple — a building in Jerusalem with three sections just like the tabernacle. Then finally with the death and resurrection of Jesus, God finished the plan that would enable him to live again in the hearts of people.

There is a definite parallel between places of worship made of brick and mortar and those made of flesh and blood. Needless to say, we tend to do a far better job keeping up our church buildings than we do our bodies. We put in marble floors, mosaic tile, original artwork, plush pews, lofty choir stands, the best woods, rich colors and tapestries, and thick carpet. We add on wings and balconies, landscape the grounds, hire a maintenance staff, and do a whole host of other things to make sure the church building looks spectacular. But there is a lot we can learn about how to take care of ourselves by studying the purpose of the tabernacle and temple, the materials used to build them, and the rules God established for preserving these structures.

Why God Set Up Earthly Dwelling Places for Himself

Before Adam and Eve's forbidden fruit snack, God walked with them in the Garden of Eden. There was no need for a special building for them to meet. At that time, nothing separated them from their Maker. God had put his spirit into Adam and Eve. That spirit was alive and well, so God connected with them on that level — Creator to creation.

After sin tainted the environment, the Bible record shows God continued to interact on some level with certain people one-on-one (e.g., Noah, Abraham, Isaac, Jacob, etc.), but the group connection was apparently missing until after the Egyptian exodus. After Moses got the Jews set free from Egyptian slavery, he went up on Mt. Sinai for forty days and forty nights (Exodus 24:18). There the Lord said to him, "Let them make Me a sanctuary, that I may dwell among them" (Exodus 25:8). While the ex-slaves were in the wilderness, God had them build the tabernacle as the physical place where he would dwell among them. Part of their honeymoon in the wilderness would be to learn through tabernacle ceremonies how to worship and interact with their God — to get to know him and relate to him on all levels: spirit, soul, and body.

They certainly needed to get to know God after over four hundred years in bondage. Their only exposure to authority had been negative for far too long. God wanted to show them love and start conditioning them to love and trust him. In the wilderness, he taught them not only how to interact with him, but also how to live with each other and how to eat and maintain their health. The tabernacle symbolized this new lifestyle. And the animal sacrifice that went on there pointed the way to the ultimate sacrifice of Jesus Christ as the perfect Lamb of God who hundreds of years later would take away the sins of the world (John 1:29).

After Israel entered the Promised Land, God directed them to fight to claim it. It took years, but once the homeland was secure, Israel's King David wanted to build a temple to the Lord to replace the tabernacle. But the Lord would not let him do it because he had been a "man of war." (1 Chronicles 28:2-3) This means he had fought as a soldier and it seems God did not want a warrior who had shed blood in battle to build his temple. Instead, he allowed David's son Solomon to build it (see 2 Chronicles 2).

When Solomon finished the temple around 965 B.C., the priests sang and praised the Lord with thanksgiving saying: "'For He is good, for His mercy endures forever,' that the house, the house of the Lord was filled with a cloud, so that the priests could not continue ministering because of the cloud; for the glory of the Lord filled the house of God. Then Solomon spoke: 'The Lord said He would dwell in the dark cloud. I have surely built you an exalted house, and a place for you to dwell in forever'" (2 Chronicles 5:13—6:1-2).

After the people brought countless sheep and oxen for sacrificing to the Lord (2 Chronicles 5:6), Solomon prayed a powerful prayer in which he put God in remembrance of his promises to King David to preserve David's royal family line. He also prayed for protection over the people of Israel. "When Solomon had finished praying, fire came down from heaven and consumed the burnt offering and the sacrifices; and the glory of the Lord filled the temple. And the priests could not enter the house of the Lord, because the glory of the Lord had filled the Lord's house" (2 Chronicles 7:1-2).

Again, God demonstrated his desire to dwell among his people and to have a special place to meet with them. Even though the priests could not enter the house while the Lord's glory was present, they were still very much aware of his visit. And that was the whole point — for them to know when God was present, to hear his voice and do his will.

Later on as the Jewish nation continued to build its history as the chosen people, God told one of their prophets he would come to dwell with all mankind in an even more intimate fashion. "And it shall come to pass afterward that I will pour out my Spirit on all flesh" (Joel 2:28). Just before his resurrection, Jesus repeated that promise. He told his disciples,

> *And I will pray the Father, and He shall give you another Comforter, that he may abide with you forever; Even the Spirit of truth; whom the world cannot receive, because it seeth him not, neither knoweth him: but ye know him; for he dwelleth with you and shall be in you. I will not leave you comfortless; I will come to you. Yet a little while, and the world seeth me no more; but ye see me; because I live, ye shall live also. At that day ye shall know that I am in my Father, and ye in me, and I in you. ~ John 14:16-20 (KJV)*

After his resurrection and before he went back to heaven, Christ said, "But you shall receive power when the Holy Spirit has come upon you" (Acts 1:8a). This happened while the disciples and other followers of Christ were meeting in a room. The Holy Spirit showed up in the form of "a rushing mighty wind" and "divided tongues, as of fire. … And they were all filled with the Holy Spirit and began to speak with other tongues, as the Spirit gave them utterance" (Acts 2:1-4). God had fulfilled his promise and set up camp in his new tabernacle — the hearts of people who believe in him!

Each of God's three dwelling places (the tabernacle, the temple, and people's hearts) had the same ultimate purpose. They were designed as a place for God's presence — the place where his Spirit would lead and guide us in all areas of our lives. It is this presence that equips us to live in the world and not be of the world. It is this presence that enables us to obey Him when our five senses tell us to do the opposite. To think that the God of the universe would lower himself to this extent so he can personally interact with us! Oh, what an incredible gift! It is almost incomprehensible.

But is your physical body fit for God to live in? The Apostle Paul throws out a similar question in his letter to the church at Corinth. He wrote, "Do you not know that you are the temple of God and that the Spirit of God dwells in you? If anyone defiles the temple of God, God will destroy him. For the temple of God is holy, which temple you are" (1 Corinthians 3:16-17).

Are you treating God's dwelling place as you should? Have you gotten rid of those things that may keep you from living out your life purpose, including unhealthy lifestyles? Do you need some encouragement? If so, then take a look at the similarities between how the tabernacle and temple were constructed and maintained as compared to how our bodies are built and should be maintained. The tabernacle and the temple were made up of three parts: the Outer Court, the Holy Place, and the Most Holy Place. Imagine a large rectangle with three sections. Just like these structures, people are made up of three parts: body, soul, and spirit.

Construction of the Tabernacle

Just as God put his best in us when we were made, he instructed the Hebrews to do the same when they built the tabernacle. It was made with their offerings. They gave up some things precious to them to build God's holy temple. They gave the wealth they took from their Egyptian enemies (see Exodus 34:4-9) — pure gold, silver and bronze, fine woven linen — and used it to build God's house. Egypt had incredible resources and only the best would do for the tabernacle.

It was built from the inside out. God had the people make the furniture first. The most important piece was the Ark of the Covenant, which was made before any of the other furniture (Exodus 25:10, 37). This object resembled a hope chest and was placed in the most sacred part of the tabernacle called the "Most Holy Place" or "Holy of Holies." It was there that God met and spoke to the Hebrew high priest and displayed his glory (Exodus 25:22). In a human temple, our spirit would be equivalent to the Most Holy Place. As Jesus said, "God is Spirit, and those who worship Him must worship in spirit and truth" (John 4:24).

Next were the furnishings for the Holy Place. This was the second area of the tabernacle between the outer court and the sacred Holy of Holies. A veil (or curtain) separated the Holy Place from the Holy of Holies. Only priests could enter the Holy Place. It was the middle part of the temple, the last place to go through before meeting God behind the veil. There, the priest offered prayers on a gold altar. The Holy Place also had a table of acacia wood, pans, pitchers, bowls, and an altar of acacia wood for incense (Exodus 25:23, 40:22). This represented mankind's soul — the place where the mind, will, emotions, intellect, and conscience reside. It is the place where decisions are made prior to going before the Lord.

Last, the Outer Court was built (Exodus 27:9). This symbolizes our physical body or flesh. As with us, it is the first thing people see. It is like the package that contains the valuable merchandise.

There are many lessons in the way God told the Hebrews to build the tabernacle. God is a God of order. He only uses the best material for his projects. He is consistent — the same yesterday, today, and forever (Hebrews 13:8). He does everything for a purpose. And he does everything for our good.

It is also interesting to note how some of the tabernacle's building materials looked similar to some of our bodies' materials and served similar purposes (see Exodus 26 and 36). For instance, the curtains for the tabernacle were made with blue, purple, and scarlet thread. These are the colors of our veins and blood vessels, which look like threads running through our bodies.

Curtains of goat hair were made for the tent over the tabernacle as our hair covers our skulls. Ram skins — dyed red — and badger skins covered the tent as our skin covers our human frame. Boards of acacia wood standing upright were used for the tabernacle walls. This is comparable to our bones. Silver sockets were used to connect the boards as our joints connect our arms, legs, hands, and feet. Could God have been giving us a message about our flesh? Were these similarities put in the Bible to teach us some spiritual *and* physical lessons?

Upgrading From the Tabernacle to the Temple

The tabernacle was later replaced with King Solomon's more upscale temple. It was laid out in the exact same order: Most Holy Place, Holy Place, and Outer Court. But Solomon's version was much fancier. The God of the desert nomads had moved to the city of Jerusalem and the temple was Solomon's grand tribute to him. Chapter two in the book of 2 Chronicles details the lengths to which Solomon went to build this temple. He organized a team of thousands of men: seventy thousand to bear burdens and eighty thousand to "quarry stone in mountains" (2 Chronicles 2:2). He sent to Hiram, the king of Tyre, for men skilled at working in gold and silver, bronze and iron, purple, crimson, and blue and who were also experienced engravers. Solomon also requested "cedar and cypress and algum logs from Lebanon," saying, "…the temple which I am about to build shall be great and wonderful" (2 Chronicles 2:9)

The temple entryway was overlaid with pure gold (2 Chronicles 3:4). The inside of the temple was also overlaid with pure gold, as was the altar (1 Kings 6:21-22). Solomon decorated the house with precious stones for beauty and overlaid the beams and doorposts, walls and doors with gold. He also carved cherubim (angels) on the walls (2 Chronicles 2:7).

The Most Holy Place was overlaid with six hundred talents of gold. In today's economy, a talent would be worth about $660,000 according to online encyclopedia Wikipedia (www.en.wikipedia.org). That equals $396 million dollars! "The weight of the nails was fifty shekels of gold; and he overlaid the upper area with gold" (2 Chronicles 2:9). One U.S. dollar today equals about four Israeli shekels. (www.en.wikipedia.org). The amount of precious metals used in that most sacred of places clearly indicate its significance to God and man.

The veil (or curtain) between the Most Holy Place and the Holy Place was of "blue, purple, crimson, and fine linen" and cherubim were woven into it (2 Chronicles 2:14). The bronze sea (large circular basin or tank), in which the priests washed, stood on twelve carved oxen and its brim was shaped like the brim of a cup, like a lily blossom (I Kings 7:23-26, Exodus 30:18-21). Ten additional bronze lavers (or basins) were made for washing the burnt offerings (I Kings 7:27 Exodus 29:31, Leviticus 8:21).

Ten lamp stands of gold were set in the temple. Ten tables were put there, too. One hundred gold bowls were made. Finally "Solomon brought in the things which his father David had dedicated: the silver and the gold and all the furnishings. And he put them in the treasuries of the house of God" (2 Chronicles 5:1). Clearly, Solomon understood what this structure represented. Only the best would do. He spared no expense.

God's Human Temples

God made man in an order similar to that used to make the tabernacle and temple. He first made man a spirit being so he would have a place to meet with him (Genesis 1:26). This is comparable to the Most Holy Place in the tabernacle and temple. Then he made his body of the dust of the earth — similar to the Outer Court. Finally, God breathed into man the breath of life or "spirit of life" as described in the Amplified Bible (Genesis 2:7). This activated man's soul which could be compared to the tabernacle's Holy Place.

In other words, God first made our spirit, the place where he would dwell in us, and then he built the outer structure or flesh. Next he breathed life or physical consciousness into man. This is why the Bible says we are "fearfully and wonderfully made" (Psalm 139:14). Science pretty much agrees with this. After thousands of years of study, many parts of the human body are still mysteries to doctors. The brain is particularly perplexing.

We have miles of blood vessels inside us. We have an amazing ability to self-heal. When we cut ourselves, our immune system immediately begins fixing the wound. Lungs blackened with coal tar from cigarettes turn pink again after people quit smoking. Our fingers are made with such precision that we can pick up a dime, play a piano, or perform delicate surgery.

Our skin is soft — yet strong enough to withstand many harsh weather conditions and keep our internal organs from harm. Our eyelashes protect our eyes from harmful foreign objects. Our backbones allow us to bend, stoop, and recline with minimal wear and tear from normal usage. Yes, we are built with incredible precision.

Only a Divine Designer could have made us. It is simply ridiculous to think, as evolution teaches, that we crawled up out of the slime as a single celled organism and grew into the complex beings we are today. No, God made us. He put the best in us and designed these temporary bodies to last for years in good health with a good quality of life. His plan is for the whole person to prosper, to be fit, and to exercise dominion in the earth, to subdue the planet and do all things to his glory.

But for some reason, we have not yet fully implemented the plan. Although Christ paid the high price and bought back everything lost in the Garden of Eden, the wonderful gift of healthy living is still not showing up consistently in the *entire* body of Christ. Part of the reason may be that we do not understand the spiritual or physical significance of blood.

Maintenance of the Tabernacle & Temple

It was noted in an earlier chapter that "The life of the flesh is in the blood" (Leviticus 17:11). We emphasize this passage again because blood was very important part of tabernacle and temple activities and it is an important part of our spiritual and physical life. The only reason the tabernacle and temple were needed in the first place was because sin earned mankind a date with death (see Genesis 2:17; Romans 6:23). Despite the presence of sin in the earth, these structures gave Holy God a way to re-connect with sinful man. The blood from animals sacrificed in the tabernacle symbolically replaced the death caused by sin with life. It was like a blood transfusion given to sick or dying people to give them new life.

Only certain animals were sacrificed in the tabernacle for their blood. It had to be perfect, without a blemish. When this animal's blood was offered to God once a year on the Day of Atonement, God pushed the sins of the Jewish people forward another year. This blood was literally their lifeline. And it was taken through every part of the temple — the Outer Court, the Holy Place, and the Holy of Holies — just as our blood flows through our entire bodies. These blood sacrifices went on for hundreds of years. They stopped in 70 A.D. after the Romans destroyed the Jewish temple in Jerusalem.

For Christians, Jesus was the perfect sacrifice. His blood redeemed us from our sins once and for all. While we are waiting for him to come back to get us, we should take very seriously how we maintain our physical temples where God dwells. Are we taking care of our bodies by only bringing in the finest materials? Are we protecting our organs, our skin, and the blood flowing through our veins? Or do we have attackers like diabetes, cancer, high cholesterol, etc., invading our territory? Our blood will usually tell the story.

Another lesson from the tabernacle/temple rituals might help us get our diets under control. First of all, *sacrifice* took place in the temple in the Outer Court — meaning you must be willing to give up or lose something in your service to God for the sake of something better. For the Jews, it was a perfect animal. For you, it might be some of your favorite foods. Next, *consecration* or cleansing took place in the temple's Holy Place. That was the purpose of the washbasin (called a bronze laver) in which the high priest would wash himself before entering the Most Holy Place. This washing symbolized that the priest had prepared his heart and was ready to meet with God and submit to his will. In order to be healthy, you have to prepare your mind to submit your lifestyle to God's will.

Finally, *offering* was made in the tabernacle behind the veil. Offering is an act of worship in which you eagerly present to God something precious and valuable to you as a way of showing your love and devotion to him. Decide now that you want to present yourself back to God as a new and improved temple.

A lot of people put on their "Sunday best" for God when they go to church. We praise God with song and dance. We invoke his power through prayer. We hear his voice through pastors and teachers. We sit up straight and put on our holy faces. Some of us clap and raise our hands in praise to God. We greet and hug our fellow believers. And in all these expressions, we use our physical bodies — even though they are sometimes tired, medicated, and struggling with diseases. Yet we still press on to come before his throne. Imagine coming before him in full health, fit in all ways for his service. You can if you start thinking like a soldier in a war and fight for your temple.

Durability of the Tabernacle & Temple

Satan is always trying to corrupt places of worship or steal their resources. He took several shots at the Jewish temple over the years before it was finally destroyed. King Nebuchadnezzar of Babylon raided it in 586 B.C., stripped it of all valuables and took the Israelites captive. Jewish patriots Ezra, Nehemiah, and Zerubbabel were allowed to return from captivity around 458 B.C., resettle Jerusalem, and restore the temple worship that had stopped after Nebuchadnezzar's raid. In 40 B.C. King Herod the Great — a master builder and egomaniac — set out to restore the temple to the glory of Solomon's day. He greatly improved the work done by the patriots. The children of Israel might not have always obeyed God in everything he told them to do, but they did understand the importance of having the temple and making sure it was the best it could be.

Jesus later predicted this structure would one day be reduced to rubble stone by stone (Matthew 24:2). And in 70 A.D. the Roman general Titus did just that by burning and destroying the temple. He then sacrificed a pig on the altar. A pig of all things! In Deuteronomy 14:8, God declared swine an unclean animal. It was not to be used in temple sacrifices or eaten by the Jews. But the defilement of God's holy site did not end with the temple destruction in 70 A.D.

In 135 A.D., Roman emperor Hadrian built a temple to Jupiter, the Greek god of love, on the land where the Jewish temple had been. Around 636 A.D., the Muslims built a mosque on the site and between 687-691 A.D. added the Dome of the Rock shrine. It and the Al Aqsa mosque stand there today in Jerusalem on what is known as the Temple Mount or Mt. Moriah. Three major religions (Jewish, Christian, and Muslim) consider the area sacred. Today, the area is Muslim controlled. Current clashes between the Jews and

Palestinians were launched when Israeli Prime Minister Ariel Sharon went to worship at that mount in 2000 during the High Holy Days. Even after millennia, it is still among the most hotly contested land on the entire planet. All sides are standing their ground and are willing to fight to defend this place where God's temple once stood.

It would be wonderful if we felt the same way about our physical temples. They symbolize the presence of God. He made sure the best was in the temple building in Jerusalem and he made sure he put the best in us. The enemy always goes after God's temples because there is great wealth in them. When they are destroyed, representations of God are destroyed. Our job is to do everything possible to make sure this does not happen. We might begin by applying some of the principles God gave the ancient Jews to keep their lives and place of worship in a manner pleasing to God.

First of all they had to strictly obey all of the guidelines by which God told them to live, including temple rituals and maintenance. Every time the Jews disobeyed or rejected God, something bad happened — either somebody died and/or the temple was destroyed. When Nebuchadnezzar raided the temple, the people had turned away from God. When Titus destroyed the temple, the majority of Jews had rejected Jesus.

In the Old Testament, the sons of Eli the priest, Hophni and Phinehas, broke the rules of the temple and paid with their lives. As priests they were entitled to a portion of the animal sacrifices for food. But Hophni and Phinehas took more than the law allowed. The law also required that the fat part of the meat first be burned by boiling it in water before the priest took his share. But Hophni and Phinehas demanded their part before the fat was burned. It was prophesied they would die for their disobedience, and they did, along with their father, Eli, who failed to correct them, and Phinehas' wife, who died in childbirth (1 Samuel 2:12-17, 27-36; 4:12-22).

The high priests, who managed to leave the Holy of Holies alive, followed the rules. They did not choose an animal God told them not to use. They did not choose a monkey as the animal for the blood sacrifice instead of a sheep. They did not get to say, "Well, instead of having shewbread on the table in the Holy Place, I'll use Lorna Doones shortbread cookies or Oreos." They followed the procedure God designed for the temple. They did not bring in anything God did not tell them to bring in. If we do likewise, the life we live in these wonderful temples God made for us will be much better.

Chapter Summary

1. God designated three places as his earthly dwellings — the tabernacle, the temple and the hearts of people.
2. He used only the best materials in all of these structures.
3. Children of God are responsible for preserving their physical temples just as the priests were responsible for preserving the wilderness tabernacle and the temple building in Jerusalem.
4. The temple is preserved when people follow God's maintenance instructions.

Kristy Dotson & Christine Tennon

Part Two

Physical Warfare

Chapter Eleven

Boot Camp

In 1918, the flu killed more people than World War I. It was
the crudest twist of fate. By the end of the war, millions
already killed in battle, over twenty million died at the hands
of a global killer, the Spanish Flu. Our war on disease is a war
we will continue to fight — until every disease is conquered.
~ Pharmaceutical company advertisement in Newsweek,
Fall/Winter 2001

Ever notice how the Bible is full of war stories and conflict? From Cain and Abel
through the early church's struggle with Roman oppression, the entire Bible is a record of
open combat followed by mighty moves of God. Why did God allow so much bickering to
go on? Was it because he was an angry God? Did he enjoy witnessing blood, sweat, and
tears? What were the people fighting over anyway? Money? Land? Power? On the surface
it was land — the best land, flowing in milk and honey. But the Jews were really fighting
to build a new culture. They were wiping out their enemies on God's order to set up a
society ruled by the Lord Almighty instead of heathen kings.

To complete this rigorous assignment, possessing the land from its paganistic
inhabitants and establishing a godly kingdom required warfare. Things are no different
today. Fortunately, God knew the children of Israel were going to have to engage in war
and he spent a great deal of time (forty years) preparing them for the series of battles
necessary to secure the Promised Land. This preparation period is detailed in the books of
Exodus, Leviticus, Numbers, and Deuteronomy; these books are a prelude to the book of
Joshua, where the battles begin.

Let's look at what happened after the Jews were liberated from Egypt as described in
Exodus. For starters, the principle of headship was established. Moses was called to
leadership and embarked on a mission to take some two to three million Israelites on a
forty-year field trip through the wilderness. Now realize at that time there was no

motorized transportation, no AAA, and no *7-Eleven* convenience stores along the way. It took order to successfully make a journey of this magnitude. Moses was the commander-in-chief for this mission, yet under the instruction of his general, the Lord God Almighty. God established lifestyle boundaries — beginning with the Ten Commandments — and the children of Israel were taught the reality of authority and submission, although they did not always obey. Nevertheless, during their forty-year journey they were repeatedly taught that in order to survive, they had to rely on God as their source for food, protection, and direction. Again, this lesson was meant to prepare them for what was yet to come.

Next, we move to the book of Leviticus. Again, the Israelites received more "basic training." Surely, they must have felt like new recruits in God's army. Here the children of Israel were taught conduct for the first time. Remember, they had been immersed in Egyptian culture for over four hundred years. The teachings of Abraham, Isaac, and Jacob were no doubt faint memories at this point. So in Leviticus, they were called to a life of holiness and separation from their worldly ways. Instead, God directed them to follow his ways. The laws of sacrifice were laid down and they were given various other codes to follow. These sacrifices, rules, and regulations were not empty rituals, but were activities designed to separate them from a sinful nature so they could establish a relationship with Holy God.

First came the laws of offerings (burnt meat, peace, sin, trespass) (Leviticus 1–7). These were sacrifices made unto the Lord. They represented his headship, his authority, and that everything first and foremost belongs to God. No battle can be won without proper leadership and God was training his people for victory by teaching them to follow him.

God's people were then taught how to eat to prepare their physical bodies to survive the wilderness and to provide strength for battle through the dietary laws. These laws were defined by the categories of "clean and unclean" foods (Leviticus 11). For health reasons, only clean animals were given the consumption green light. Unclean animals were an abomination. Laws related to physical cleanliness were next (Leviticus 12–15) followed by the law regarding the Day of Atonement (Leviticus 16), laws on special sacrifices (Leviticus 17), laws about unlawful sexual conduct (Leviticus 18), and personal conduct laws such as keeping the Sabbath, idol worship, stealing, lying, fraud, unrighteous judgment, gossiping, vengeance, etc. (Leviticus 19).

As we journey into the book of Numbers, we see another stage in the preparation process. For the first time since he left Egypt, Moses had to take inventory and determine exactly how many people of God would be able to fight in Canaan. With the exclusion of the tribe of Levi, Moses organized his troops into twelve tribes, of which he had a force of 603,550 (Numbers 1:21-43). They were assembled around the "Tabernacle of Meeting," which no doubt looked like a military campground, similar to the Pentagon. It was in this traveling camp that God dwelt and from which he, through Moses, gave the people their marching orders to fight. The orders given were an "all or nothing" assignment where there would be no turning back once the plan for taking Canaan was put in motion:

> *And the Lord spake unto Moses in the plains of Moab by Jordan near Jericho, saying, "Speak unto the children of Israel, and say unto them, When ye are passed over Jordan into the land of Canaan; Then ye shall drive out all the inhabitants of the land from before you, and destroy all their pictures, and destroy all their molten images, and quite pluck down all their high places. And ye shall dispossess the inhabitants of the land, and dwell therein: for I have given you the land to possess it." ~ Numbers 33:50-53 (KJV)*

Sounds like a tough assignment, huh? But aren't all military assignments that involve conflict tough? God's people had to be ready, for the time had come for them to put up or shut up. Before they entered Canaan, Moses passed his leadership mantle on to Joshua. "And Joshua the son of Nun was full of the spirit of wisdom; for Moses had laid his hands upon him: and the children of Israel hearkened unto him, and did as the Lord commanded Moses" (Deuteronomy 34:9 KJV),

Moses laid his hands on Joshua for the sole purpose of transferring the spirit of wisdom so Joshua could lead the people. Again, this was yet another step in the preparation process: responsibility. From that point forward, Joshua duplicated what he had been taught by getting his newly acquired troops ready for battle. "We're going into battle. Get ready! Get ready! Get ready!" was probably the unexpected announcement Joshua made three days before his troops began their journey into Canaan. He commanded the officers of the people, "Pass through the camp and command the people, saying, 'Prepare provisions for yourselves, for within three days you will cross over this Jordan, to go in to possess the land which the Lord your God is giving you to possess' " (Joshua 1:11). Again, more preparation. Only this time, the preparation period was reduced from forty years to seventy-two hours. After forty years in the wilderness, and the daily instructions directly from the Lord, God expected his people to be ready to fight, win, and reign. And they did.

Now ask yourself, how prepared are we today to live a full, productive, and purposeful life knowing much of it hinges on how well we are physically? How ready are we as a church body? How ready are you personally? Are you spiritually prepared? With all the preaching and Bible teaching programs on the air, and the books, tapes, CDs, and DVDs available, you probably are. Christians are taught how to recite Scripture to get through each day and protect themselves from the works of the enemy. We are taught that the Word of God must serve as our daily bread, feeding our hearts with the ammunition needed to deflect any bullet Satan or his army may fire at us. This daily dose of God's written Word is our source of encouragement, protection, and shield.

Since life and death lie in the power of our tongues, we use our mouths as weapons of warfare as well. Weekly, if not daily, we go into our bomb shelters, or prayer closets, and confess the outcome we expect before we go into battle. If we feel the struggle is much larger than expected, we resort to Plan B, pulling in the "big guns." This is when we get on the telephone and call our fellow Christian prayer warriors. They have no problem meeting the enemy head on, or face-to-face, engaging in full-fledged battle by interceding and paving the way for our victory. Spiritual warfare is essential. Because the enemy is lurking about in an unseen realm, and because we are speaking spirits, the battle against him must be carried out first in the invisible realm before the results we want can show up in the natural world.

Now, let me ask, "Are you physically prepared for war"? Uh-oh, I may have stepped on a toe or two. You don't have to answer. You already know. All too often emphasis is placed solely on the spiritual component and not the physical aspect of warfare. Let's bring some balance to Christian warfare. Just like in the army, physical strength is required to carry the artillery and defeat the enemy. Since the land of Canaan was no small backyard, Joshua and his armed forces had to travel hundreds of miles during a twenty-five-year period. They had to be in excellent physical condition. Joshua covered all the bases. He was spiritually well-grounded for he had to be able to hear from the Lord at all times and he demonstrated his physical agility as he bypassed retirement and worked until he died at age 110. So even in his latter years, Joshua was in shape to do battle for God. God had mandated he "be strong and of good courage" (Joshua 1:9), and so he was.

According to *Webster's Ninth New Collegiate Dictionary*, the word *strong* has several definitions suitable in describing Joshua and his team of soldiers:

1. Having or marked by great physical power
2. Not mild or weak
3. Having moral or intellectual power
4. Having great resources (as of wealth or talent)
5. Not easily injured or disturbed.

This definition describes both the spiritual (intangible) *and* physical attributes of a strong person. So, if physical strength is important for battle, why are so many Christians on the battlefield of life without it? Because we have not made it a priority, plain and simple. God's representatives should be physically fit and stand out favorably in the crowd. As Joshua was preparing to fight his first battle in Jericho, he encountered a representative of God's army who was *very* noticeable. Initially, Joshua thought the man may have been his enemy, but his attire and demeanor was of the Holy One.

> *And it came to pass, when Joshua was by Jericho, that he lifted up his eyes and looked, and, behold, there stood a man over against him with his sword drawn in his hand: and Joshua went unto him, and said unto him, Art thou for us, or for our adversaries? And he said, Nay; but as captain of the host of the Lord am I now come. And Joshua fell on his face to the earth, and did worship, and said unto him, What saith my lord unto his servant? ~ Joshua 5:13-14 (KJV)*

This high-ranking servant was distinguished. His drawn sword indicated he was ready. What message is conveyed to the public when you are met on the street? Does your body language say, "I am a walking example of the picture of perfect health that our Lord has promised to all believers"? Or does your extra weight and slow-paced walk blow your cover and cause you to merely blend in with the rest of the sick and challenged world? How the world views you is a strong indicator of how well they will receive the Gospel.

The U.S. armed forces are highly effective in recruiting new members to their organizations because of the image portrayed in their advertising campaigns. You will never see an unfit soldier as the poster child for the Marines. Instead, you typically see an attractive, clean-cut, and physically fit man or woman all dressed up in military attire. Their uniforms are neatly pressed and as they stand at attention the message written on their faces says they are engaged in serious business. Now if God's business is such a serious matter, which it is, then all Christians must be representatives of God's best.

God is sending out his battle cry to his people. He is telling us to stop using external adornment (St. John, Armani, and Prada suits) to cover up the physical evidence of our poor eating habits and failure to exercise. Having cute saints on Sunday and ineffective saints Monday through Saturday is not what God desires. He would much rather we tend to the cells, tissues, muscles, organs, and organ systems he has given us to keep our bodies functioning at peak capacity. We should bypass the cover-ups and the short- cuts and prepare ourselves to do kingdom business by following Paul's direction and put on the entire armor of God. We should be equipped in all areas for his work, inside and out.

A component of preparation is submitting to military indoctrination, which involves a bit of mind renewal. The children of Israel went through this process while in the wilderness. They were exposed to new levels of authority, conduct, rules, and responsibility. When enlisted and called to action, new recruits to the armed forces must do the same. A soldier must accept his commitment to the armed forces, make a decision to convert to military protocol, and accept and obey the commands of his officers. There is no way around it.

Rebellion within the ranks of authority can be costly, whereas submission can lead to safety and security. What path the new recruit decides to take is entirely up to him since he will bear the consequences. His submission is determined by his attitude, and his obedience to authority is a matter of conduct. If the soldier does not fall in line, his disobedience will not only have a negative effect on him but also on the lives and mission of the entire unit.

Consider yourself a new recruit in God's army. Before you can serve on the front lines you have to endure boot camp, where your initial transformation begins. Both your mind and your body will be renewed. Your first assignment?

1. Accept where you are. Admit to yourself your health and physique are not up to par. Agree you may not have been taking the best care of your body and the time has come for you to change. Like a new recruit enlisting, create a contract with yourself and sign your name, holding yourself accountable for your commitment to change.

2. Make a decision to live differently. For things to change, you must change. To get a different result, you have to do something different. Make a decision that you are going to control your destiny by adopting a new, healthier lifestyle. If your daily schedule does not include an exercise program, start one. Too tired to workout

after work? Then rearrange your schedule so you get up an hour earlier to squeeze in a workout during the morning. If you routinely eat out in restaurants five days a week, make a decision that at least three nights you will cook at home. Your initial weeks of adopting a healthy lifestyle will be a challenge, yet you will become conditioned to the new routine with time.

3. Accept truth and correction. Constantly seek the truth and guidance from experts for maintaining your health. Various resources are available to you. Recognize the truth (advice) may sound foreign to you and may be different from what you have been taught in the past. Know that the truth you know (and apply) will make you free. Receive "healthful" information with gladness and without resistance.

Whether you like it or not, you are in the military now: the Lord's military. It is necessary to submit everything you are to him for kingdom refinement. Your thoughts, your habits, your time, your money, and, yes, your flesh. There is a hefty price to pay if you don't. Life in the kingdom of God is a progressive walk. It starts with a decision to get ready — spiritually and physically. We should not turn back and those who are A.W.O.L need to return to active duty immediately. We must prepare ourselves physically for our God-given assignments, and do everything necessary to live long enough to complete them. Every hand is needed, for the fight is on and it is intensifying. The good news is we have a General in charge who has never lost a battle and never will.

Chapter Summary

1. Physical warfare goes hand in hand with spiritual warfare when it comes to good health.
2. Physical warfare entails preparing the body by strengthening it with proper food and exercise.
3. Before engaging in physical warfare, you must first renew your mind and:
   3.1. Come to terms with your present health status.
   3.2. Make a commitment to a lifestyle change for the benefit of your health.
   3.3. Be open to receiving new truths and "healthful" information.

Chapter Twelve

Counting the Costs

Now a certain woman had a flow of blood for twelve years,
and had suffered many things from many physicians. She
had spent all that she had and was no better, but rather grew
worse. ~ Mark 5:25-26

Poor health is expensive. It can rob people of money in a lot of different ways. It can steal peace of mind. It can imprison people in their homes, in hospitals, or in nursing care facilities. It can destroy relationships. Then after stripping away things important to a good life, it delivers the final blow. Poor health will kill you if you let it.

The woman in the Mark 5 passage above was believed to have suffered from "female problems." Some disease or condition in her reproductive organs might have caused her abnormal bleeding. Maybe she had fibroid tumors in her womb, which can cause long and painful menstrual cycles. Whatever it was, this medical condition cost her *all* her money as she tried to get well and "suffered many things from many physicians." Still, they could not help her.

It also may have interfered with her social life. According to Old Testament laws, "If a woman has a discharge, and the discharge from her body is blood, she shall be set apart seven days; and whoever touches her shall be unclean until evening" (Leviticus 15:19). Anyone who sat or laid on anything on which she had sat or lain was considered unclean. So it is possible this woman was isolated from her husband (if she had one), isolated from other family members, and isolated from people in her community. Maybe she was not even touched or hugged during her twelve-year ordeal. Back in those days, no one wanted to be declared "unclean." If you were labeled unclean you had to wash your clothes, bathe in water, and be "unclean until evening" (Leviticus 15:21). You were socially alienated, which could be embarrassing.

The reasons for these laws were probably practical as well as symbolic. God gave them to Moses while the Jews were living in the wilderness after they left Egypt. There were thousands of people in that desert and good sanitation was important to keep them alive. The laws also symbolized mankind's spiritual condition. They taught these ex-slaves how sin can separate them from Holy God and prevent them from having the relationship with Him that God intended from the beginning. These rules and regulations — some of which seem odd to us today — reminded them daily that there was a price to be paid for sin, and only God could cleanse them.

The Mosaic Law was still in effect during the time this woman in Mark 5 was living. So here she was — sick, broke, and desperate. She was at a turning point. She was ready for a change. She had nothing else to lose.

Fast forward to our lifetime. At what point are you in this battle for good health? What have you lost? What's up for grabs next? The news headlines paint a bleak picture about the costs associated with poor health. People are paying high prices in a variety of different ways: financially (e.g., unaffordable health insurance, medical bills, lost income, day to day living expenses, etc.), emotionally, and physically. Let's look at some of the costs that are driven, to a large extent, by lifestyle choices that typically cause people to be overweight and sick with nutrition-related diseases.

Medical/Insurance Costs

U.S. healthcare spending reached $1.9 trillion in 2004. The rise has been attributed to increasing hospital and drug costs. According to the National Coalition on Health Care, the cost is expected to reach $2.9 trillion in 2009 and $4 trillion by 2015 or 20 percent of the gross national product. In 2004, the U.S. Surgeon General estimated public health costs attributable to people being overweight or obese totaled about $117 billion a year — fast approaching the $140 billion stemming from smoking.

Under our current system, some people have health insurance through their employers. But the price of this coverage has been rising every year. Employee contributions to these plans are going up and up. Some employer contributions have gone up almost three times in one year. But little is done about what's really driving these costs. Everyone just complains someone should do something. The boss should do something. The government should do something. The doctor should do something. But what about the patient?

You might feel that whether or not people take care of themselves is a private matter. But it's not. Frequent medical treatments drive up health insurance costs for everybody. There are some people who go to the doctor every month for conditions that would go away with regular exercise and healthy eating. We've all heard a relative, friend, or co-worker make complaints such as, "I'm tired" or "I have a headache" or "My stomach is upset a lot lately." Do you sympathize and say, "Ahhh! You poor thing! You should go to the doctor." Or do you ask, "What have you been eating? Have you been exercising?" Do you tell them the baby back ribs they're chowing down on might be the cause of their problem?

We all know people who eat fast food for lunch every day, gulp down four to six sodas with a cup or two of coffee in between, frequently raid the vending machines at work, and never pass up the cakes, cookies, and pies offered during on-the-job celebrations. When they get sick and go to the doctor, the cost of their treatment impacts employee and employer health plan costs, which are driven by the number of claims employees make each year. So what starts out as a personal choice could end up hitting everybody in the pocket book. One way or the other, we all end up paying for other people's poor lifestyle choices.

Author Nicholas Webb addresses this in his book, *The Cost of Being Sick*: "According to a recent study by RAND on the ill effects of our fast food, super-sized lifestyles, the way we live is directly attributable to the skyrocketing costs of health care. The study reported obesity is associated with a 36 percent increase in inpatient and outpatient expenditures and a 77 percent increase in medication. The study reinforced growing concerns about how dramatically increasing rates of obesity in the U.S. will negatively affect health-care costs as well as overall public health."

Webb says over $600 billion is spent annually on the administrative costs of health care in the United States. That is the paper-pushing part of medicine — not the treatment that carries its own hefty price tag. Webb is a medical product inventor who says rising healthcare costs will continually force businesses to pass along the increases to employees in order to protect profits. He predicts a time is coming when individuals will be 100 percent responsible for all of their health care costs. Webb calls these costs the "new mortgages," wherein healthcare bills could be over $1,000 a month for someone with an annual salary of $40,000. Furthermore, according to Webb, the ability to get coverage and what people pay will be based on their physical condition:

> Much like our current credit scoring system today, Americans will soon be "rated" by health-care insurers on the level of their health — good or bad. Factors comprising the score's formula will include medical history, genetic-risk factors, occupation, age, gender, race, body fat, and many other

personal health-related factors. A high or "good health" score will send you to the front of the line for health-care insurance. A low score, however, may result in denied access to health-care coverage. Soon we'll see Americans fretting about their "health ratings" every bit as much as they do over their credit ratings and driving records. Not only will health insurers use health scores to gauge your health risk levels, but also employers and bankers will use them to calculate your long-term employability and financial stability. ... We already have a "health score" model in life insurance and can expect to see richer data being used in the makeup of these health scores. ... In the future, we will see insurance companies rewarding individuals through HVS — Health Value Score — programs. Through such programs, coverage premiums will be based on health scores, health insurance utilization and other factors including wellness program participation and improvement from health base line. Patients will receive a refund or pay a penalty based on usage and health scores. American families will begin to look at their HVS ratings with the same interest and intensity they view their tax returns.

Webb's predictions are apparently coming to pass. The September 25, 2004 edition of the *Wall Street Journal* included an article entitled "HMOs Try 'Frequent Jogger Points.' " The subtitle read "Rewards for Participation in Healthy Activities Range from Trips to Low Co-Pays." The first sentence of the story makes a powerful point. The reporter, Johanna Bennett, wrote: "It just doesn't pay to be a couch potato." Bennett goes on:

In an effort to pry their members out of their seats and into healthier lifestyles, an increasing number of health plans are offering everything from health-club memberships to European vacations for those who exercise, lose weight, or quit smoking.

Bennett notes one company that has launched a program called "Health Credits," which awards points to participants whenever they engage in healthy activities and lets them trade in the points for everything from free exercise equipment to insurance premium discounts or lower co-payments for visits to the doctor. One health care consultant quoted in the article called these incentive programs "the wave of the future."

If you are still skeptical about Webb's dire prediction, take note of some other news headlines in recent years reporting factors that drive our current healthcare crisis:

The Centers for Disease Control report U.S. companies spend approximately $13 billion a year in health, life, and disability insurance payments and sick days, which total a loss of 39 million lost workdays annually. ~ Chicago Tribune, October 6, 2006

Premiums for employer-based health insurance rose by 7.7 percent in 2006. ~ National Coalition on Health Care

Nearly forty-seven million Americans do not have health insurance. Medical bills now rank as a top cause of personal bankruptcy in the U.S. ~ Parade Magazine, May 9, 2004

Between 1998 and 2003, employee contributions to health insurance doubled while employer's contributions rose about 60 percent. ~ Chicago Tribune, October 12, 2003

A study by the Kaiser Family Foundation and Health Research and Educational Trust reports health insurance premiums increased 11.2 percent in 2004. That's five times faster than inflation and salaries for American workers. Premiums rose by double digits for the fourth consecutive year. ~ Chicago Tribune, September 10, 2004

Some corporate retirees are seeing a cutback in their health benefits. Ten percent of the 408 companies surveyed had stopped offering the benefits to retiring employees and 20 percent said they would do so in about three years due to rapidly rising health care costs. ~ USA Today, January 15, 2004

Medicare is discarding its declaration that obesity is not a disease. This change could open the door for millions of overweight Americans to have weight loss treatment including stomach surgery covered under the program. ~ Associated Press, July 16, 2004

It is estimated people with chronic diseases account for more than two-thirds of the nation's $1.6 trillion medical bill. Disease management firms hope to cut these costs by educating patients on how to manage their symptoms so as to avoid things such as kidney failure and amputations. As baby boomers age, this number is expected to increase. ~ Wall Street Journal, October 20, 2004

The American Association of Retired Persons reported prices for name-brand medicines commonly used by seniors rose faster than inflation in the last four years. The AARP found an average price increase of 27.6 percent compared with a 10.4 percent inflation rate. ~ USA Today, May 26, 2004

Senior citizens advocacy group AARP took out a full-page ad in the Chicago Tribune urging U.S. senators to pass a bill allowing drug imports from Canada. These imported drugs cost less than they do in the U.S. ~ Chicago Tribune, July 16, 2004

Judith Stern, a nutrition professor at the University of California at Davis says the U.S. government spent $327 million on obesity research in 2003 but shelled out "a billion on cancer and AIDS research, more than a billion on heart

disease research and almost a billion on diabetes." Stern advocates that at least that much be spent on obesity.
~ Chicago Tribune, January 25, 2004

At least $2.3 billion dollars. That's the national price tag placed on the hours certain cancer patients spend sitting in doctor's waiting rooms or receiving chemotherapy during the first year of treatment. This information was part of a study published by the Journal of the National Cancer Institute. The study estimates the hours lost during the first year to cancer care include: 368 for ovarian cancer, 272 for lung cancer, and 193 for kidney cancer. The monetary value on this time is $15.23 an hour. ~ USA Today, January 3, 2007

These facts paint a sobering picture and have generated a lot of talk about how to solve the problems. A number of employers are taking action. To help lower health insurance costs, some companies are giving employees cash to lose or maintain weight. Others have stopped serving high-fat foods at workplace meetings. If you want chips with your sandwich instead of a carrot, you have to ask. One company is offering healthier food at cheaper prices in its cafeteria. A slice of pizza costs twice as much as a veggie wrap. If this trend continues, eating "comfort food" might not be so comfortable for your wallet.

The government is also making some attempts to raise public awareness of the health crisis by using media announcements to promote exercise and healthy eating since seven out of ten Americans reportedly do not exercise regularly. Money is driving this care and concern. An article in the May 14, 2003 edition of *USA Today* reported research findings published online in an issue of Health Affairs which indicated that overweight Americans cost the nation $93 billion in annual medical bills. According to the federally funded project, the government pays about half of that amount. The study also compared the medical costs for overweight and obese people with those for people of normal weight. Here is what they found:

- Overall, annual medical costs for an obese person are 37.7 percent more or $732 higher than the costs for someone of normal weight.

- An obese recipient of Medicare costs $1,486 more a year than one of healthy weight.

- An obese patient on Medicaid costs $864 more than a normal weight Medicaid recipient.

Commenting on the study, health economist Eric Finkelstein said, "The fact that Medicaid and Medicare, and ultimately taxpayers, are financing half the cost lends credence to the notion that obesity is not solely a personal issue."

Legal Costs

Some lawyers agree with this. They say it's a "corporate responsibility" issue and food makers should pay up. Obesity litigation is their new cash cow — kind of like tobacco litigation was a few years ago. The defendants are typically food manufacturers and sellers of fast foods.

One of the most famous cases was the 2002 million-dollar suit filed against McDonald's by two Bronx teenagers in New York federal court. They claimed the food chain was selling high-fat meals with unknown ingredients that made them obese and contributed to their health problems. The judge dismissed the suit, stating the accusations were legally insufficient. He also said everyone should know eating too much fast food is bad for them and "it is not the place of the law to protect (plaintiffs) from their own excesses." In 2005, the judge let the attorneys re-file the suit to try to establish the existence of dangers in McDonald's food that are "not commonly well known."

In February 2006, a class action suit was being prepared for filing in Massachusetts against soft drink manufacturers. It claims sodas are contributing to childhood obesity and it is aimed at getting the drinks out of public schools. Those pushing this litigation accuse soft drink makers of negligence and violation of consumer protection laws. At some point, the states might enter this dispute to try to recover medical costs associated with obesity, just as they did with tobacco litigation. Americans spend about $105 billion a year on fast food. These are some serious profits, and the industry will not give up a cut of that cash to plaintiffs and trial lawyers without a fight.

In 2003, A San Francisco lawyer sued Kraft Foods, seeking to stop the marketing of Oreos to children. He dropped the suit three days later, claiming Kraft told him the company planned to eliminate trans-fats from the cookie. Adding hydrogen to vegetable oil makes trans-fats. They help make food stay fresh longer and give baked goods that yummy taste we all love. They also clog arteries. Two months later, Kraft announced its launch of an anti-obesity initiative wherein it would reduce portion sizes and change the manufacturing process to make certain foods healthier.

While the public might be offended by such lawsuits and see them as justification for more lawyer jokes, some of these cases do have social significance. Yes, there are lawyers who just want to make a buck on the backs of the obese. But there are also those who want to raise public awareness and send a message to companies inclined to package anything and sell it to consumers to make a fast dollar — even if it's unhealthy. The threat of huge monetary verdicts makes these organizations sit up, take notice, and, in some instances, try to make their food products healthier.

Meantime, the U.S. House of Representatives in 2004 passed a bill (the so-called "cheeseburger bill") to ban obesity-related lawsuits against restaurants and food manufacturers. Representative Lamar Smith of Texas reportedly said, "We should not encourage lawsuits that blame others for our own choices and could bankrupt an entire industry." (http://www.cbsnews.com/2100-500368_162-956858.html). The bill did not pass the Senate but some states have passed similar legislation. (http://www.webmd/diet/news/20051019).

Now New York City has added a new dimension to what some call "nanny laws" that try to force people to eat better. In December 2006, the Big Apple's city council voted to ban all trans-fats from the food served in city restaurants. New York City restaurants must begin frying with oil that leaves food with less than half a gram of trans-fat per serving. If not, they could face fines of up to $200 per infraction starting in July 2007.

The legal fallout from lifestyle-related health problems goes beyond food and beverage manufacturers. I (Christine) was talking to an attorney friend who told me about a case he was handling involving an obese woman and a wheelchair. He represented the company that provides skycap and airport wheelchair service to airline passengers. In this particular case, the passenger was a woman who weighed over three hundred pounds. She was in a hurry to get to her gate. She was on her way to the Mayo Clinic for treatment of a variety of health problems. A wheelchair was ordered to take her to her gate.

When a young male employee arrived with a regular chair, he recommended he call back and order the Galaxy chair used for obese customers. She told him she did not have time to wait for the Galaxy so she managed to get into the smaller chair and off they went. On the way, she fell out of the chair because the seat belt was not long enough to buckle her in. Several people had to help the young man get her back into the chair. As a result of this incident, the woman sued the young man's employer for negligence over the injuries she says she sustained in the fall. Part of the claim involves a complaint that she should have been belted into the chair.

In early 2004, an Illinois couple sued the U.S. government for preventing them from buying cheaper prescription drugs from Canada. The couple claim their right to privacy was violated because of a U.S. law that prohibits the re-importation of drugs meant for sale outside America and also bans the importation of foreign-made drugs not approved by the U.S. Food & Drug Administration. The retired couple, who thought they would be living their golden years together enjoying their children and grandchildren, say the husband was forced to take a part-time job at Wal-Mart to help pay their $800 a month prescription medication bill.

Who pays for all this litigation and the changes that come afterward? Everybody. Companies consider it a cost of doing business and are covered by insurance. They then pass the cost on to consumers. The government considers it the cost of running a government and raises taxes. Again, everybody ends up paying.

Social Costs

There was an uproar a few years ago when airlines began charging overweight passengers higher fares. It was an awkward moment for the carriers and the affected customers. Thin passengers felt guilty but admitted in news reports that they cringe when they see an overweight person seated on their row of a plane — especially if it's a long flight.

In a November 24, 2006, article posted at Forbes.com, entitled "The Hidden Cost of Obesity," obesity researcher David Allison says, "Obese people are less likely to be given jobs, they're waited on more slowly, they're less likely to be given apartments, they're less likely to be sent to college by their parents." Researchers also report obese people may find it more difficult to marry or get promotions or plum job assignments than thinner people. Such discrimination is often driven by concerns about the health of obese and overweight people, as well as society's worship of anything thin.

Opera singer Deborah Voight can attest to this. In 2003, she was dismissed from the London Royal Opera because she was thought to be too large (350 pounds at one point) for a little black dress considered essential to a production. Since that time, she has had weight-loss surgery. As of October 2006, she had lost about 200 pounds and was preparing for the lead role in *Salome* — the Bible story about King Herod's stepdaughter whose seductive dance cost John the Baptist his head. This talented artist was not being shunned for her singing but for her size. Unfortunately, sometimes talent has nothing to do with it.

Personal Economic Costs

Aside from higher medical expenses, there is not much published information on what obesity related illness costs individuals; however, their life insurance premiums are reportedly two to four times as large. In general, poor health takes a financial toll on the whole family when a loved one is sick. A source of income may be lost. Living arrangements sometimes have to change. An in-law may have to move in. Perhaps a second mortgage is necessary. Medicine and/or medical equipment not paid for by the government or insurance have to be bought. Nurses are hired or a spouse or child has to quit a job and perhaps move across the country to attend to the sick relative.

Day by day, poor health eats away at our bank accounts. A newspaper ad for a treadmill sums it up nicely:

Open heart surgery	$100,000
Quadruple bypass	$75,000
Angioplasty	$50,000
Deluxe funeral	$25,000
Vision Fitness treadmill	$1,200

Instead of saving thousands of dollars on healthcare by buying a treadmill, too many people opt for the high-end fix, surgery, and/or death. The sick and shut-in continue to deplete their resources — or those of their family members — to combat some conditions that are preventable with discipline and self-control at a fraction of the cost of surgery.

Emotional Costs

I (Christine) had an uncle who left a terrible void in the family when he died from multiple health problems (including leukemia, diabetes, and high blood pressure). I'd watched him for years eat whatever he wanted despite what the doctors said. When he died, he was survived by a wife of over fifty years and nine children who adored him. He also left my aunt short on funds.

My mother's situation was different but had its own special price tag. Before my father departed this life in April 2007, she was housebound for about six years, taking care of him. He was confined to bed with severe rheumatoid arthritis and a heart condition. Mom spent her days feeding, bathing, and dressing dad with occasional assistance from home healthcare workers and various family members. Sometimes the situation got pretty stressful.

Add another patient to the roster and the pressure grows. I (Christine) have a brother, Frank, who became the other patient at one point. At the chronological age of fifty-two, he was still in his teenaged rebellion years. He did whatever he wanted to do, including letting his health get bad. He almost treated it like a badge of honor — something to brag about. At Thanksgiving, he used a platter. Not to serve the turkey, but for his holiday meal. He ate fried foods virtually every day — and lots of it. Catfish, chicken, vegetables swimming in grease, pork, spaghetti — you name it. Eventually he was diagnosed with hypertension.

One day in 2004, Frank was rushed to the hospital after having a stroke. There was bleeding on the brain. The doctors wanted to operate but initially could not figure out exactly where he was bleeding. For a while, he could not walk. My mother was not only worried about his health but about how she was going to be able to take care of him *and* my father. Fortunately, Frank made a decent recovery. But his lifestyle, including his eating habits, did not change much and my mother continued to worry. Frank's second stroke added to her concerns. Again he pulled through but his steps are a lot slower and his memory is not what it used to be.

Ultimate Costs

Excess weight is said to be the cause of up to 400,000 early deaths each year in the United States. According to a life expectancy analysis published by the *New England Journal of Medicine* in March 2005, obesity could shorten the average lifespan of an entire generation — today's children — by two to five years. The report also says obesity now reduces life expectancy by four to nine months. "Childhood obesity is like a massive tsunami headed toward the United States," said pediatric endocrinologist David Ludwig, director of the obesity program at Children's Hospital in Boston and one of the study's authors, in a March 2005 *USA Today* article. (For more on the issue of childhood obesity, see Chapter 14: Casualties of War.)

Then there are the costs associated with our quick-fix approach to fitness and weight loss. A forty-one year old Massachusetts woman and her eight-month fetus died eighteen months after she had gastric bypass surgery. According to news reports, doctors doing emergency surgery found most of the woman's small intestine had slid through a tear in an adjacent membrane. Doctors say this is a defect sometimes left after the intestines are rearranged in the bypass operation. Gangrene set in after the hole choked off blood to the stretch of intestines, and by then the fetus had died. Doctors now warn women not to get pregnant too soon after having this surgery.

A New Jersey woman featured in an August 2004 *Time* cover story, "When Fat Cells Attack," at one time weighed as much as 420 pounds. The story said she became really desperate after her left leg was amputated below the knee for complications from diabetes. She could not run, swim, or play with her child, and ended up in a wheelchair. She eventually lost 230 pounds but resorted to gastric bypass surgery to do it.

Is this procedure God's best? More and more people are opting to have it. They lose a lot of weight and feel better about themselves. However, it is heartbreaking to think of the lengths to which they felt they had to go to get to their desired weight. There is a story being told about a woman who actually <u>gained</u> weight so that she could meet the weight required for her to have this surgery.

Make a list right now of what poor health has cost or is costing you and your family. Think of how God would rather you had spent that money you used for medication. Think of what he would like to see you do with that time spent traveling to the doctor, going to the pharmacy, sitting, or confined to bed because you or a loved one is sick. Think of the energy used caring for yourself or an ailing family member. Think about the tears shed, the sleepless nights, the worry, the hospital stays, the depressing doctor's reports, and the missed opportunities to live the life you always wanted to live.

Think about God's promises, the plan he has for your life and, if you have children, your children's lives. Think about hearing him say, "Well done, good and faithful servant." Think about it and make a decision that will make the Master proud of you. Count the cost and choose to live each day as a good steward over your health. That woman with the issue of blood counted the costs and made a better decision.

> ***When she heard about Jesus, she came behind Him in the crowd and touched His garment. For she said, "If only I may touch His clothes, I shall be made well." Immediately the fountain of her blood was dried up, and she felt in her body that she was healed of the affliction. ~ Mark 5:27-29***

She had tried conventional medicine. She had followed the rules of her time. She had gone with the "norm." She had spent all she had on the world's medicines. She no doubt counted the cost of continuing her life with a "flow of blood." At that point, she had a choice to make — continue to drag through life with the status quo until she died, or try Jesus and be made well.

I (Christine) do not know what caused her condition. I do not know if it was her diet or Satan or both. I do not know how the rest of her days were after she was made whole. But I do know this woman changed her mind and changed her life. Her action was significant enough for two of Jesus' disciples (Mark and Matthew) to include her story in their gospels. This woman took a bold step and got a big reward. We should all be encouraged by her outcome and make every effort to grab and keep the health miracle God extends to us.

Chapter Summary

1. Poor health is expensive and everybody ends up paying for it.
2. U.S. healthcare spending reached $1.9 trillion in 2004 and is expected to go up another 50 percent by 2009.
3. The state of un-health in America is undermining the quality of personal and family life, generating litigation similar to the tobacco lawsuits, and ultimately killing those we love.
4. Each person has to weigh the cost of his or her own lifestyle choices and pursue the health and wholeness the bible says is available to us through faith in Jesus Christ.

Stories from the Front Lines...

The Price of One Woman's Hospital Bill Could Include Jail

A twenty-eight-year-old Illinois woman was accused of fraudulently obtaining $37,000 worth of medical treatment. She allegedly underwent gall bladder surgery using another person's health insurance card. ~ Chicago Tribune, April 29, 2004

Funeral Home Donates Custom-Made Coffin

A funeral home donated a custom-made coffin for the remains of a 48 year-old woman who died from congestive heart failure weighing 545 pounds. Her 42-inch casket — which had to be special ordered — cost four times as much as a regular sized coffin and had to be carried by twelve pallbearers versus the usual six. The mortuary donated the coffin because the woman's family had no money to pay for their services. ~ As told by a funeral director to another customer

Chapter Thirteen

Weapons of Warfare

Wherefore do ye spend money for that which is not bread? and your labour for that which satisfieth not? hearken diligently unto me, and eat ye that which is good, and let your soul delight itself in fatness. ~ Isaiah 55:2 (KJV)

Take five minutes and ponder this question. Why indeed would we spend our money on something that is not bread? In this context, "bread" should be viewed as any food item that brings nourishment to the body. So the question is why are we spending all of our precious money on food that is not feeding the body, nor bringing satisfaction to our internal hunger centers.

The question must be asked of every person, and particularly every Christian, each time he or she enters a grocery store. In nine out of ten grocery carts, you will see milk, cheese, white bread, cookies, chips, microwave meals, soda, and ice cream. It's rare to see someone at the checkout counter with a cart loaded with fruit, vegetables, whole grain bread, and purified water. The sad reality is many people think they are pretty good at shopping for healthy foods. But they are not. They have been led to believe that if an item is in the grocery store and the federal government has approved it for sale, then it must be safe for consumption. They think that food wrapped in a fancy, brightly colored package with "natural" printed on it, can't possibly do them any harm. Guess again. I (Kristy) used to believe this nonsense as well.

After I finished graduate school in 1991, I began an eight-year career in the processed foods industry. Armed with a background in engineering, I was on course to become extensively involved with the process of taking a food product from the idea stage through manufacturing. I was excited, as my schooling was behind me and I was equipped to do my part in "feeding America." What a fool I was. Later on, I began to feel as if I was doing my part in killing America. I spent several years working for some of the top food companies in the world — General Mills and Kraft Foods. I even took a tour through the fast food industry by working for a company called Perseco, which was the procurement arm of packaging materials for McDonald's. Over time, certain experiences I had working in this industry alerted me that there was something terribly wrong with our U.S. food system.

The first warning came one summer when, while working in quality control, I witnessed an entire department turn into complete pandemonium as they were forced to quarantine fifty million boxes of cereal and fifteen bushels of raw oats. This decision was the result of discovering cereal was being sold that contained traces of an unauthorized pesticide not approved for use on stored oats. The cereal had been selling for thirteen months before it was discovered during a routine test by FDA inspectors. This meant consumers had undoubtedly eaten some of the cereal in the contaminated packages.

Here I was working in "quality control," yet I was helpless as I watched my co-workers work overtime to resolve the matter. As attorney after attorney entered our department to meet with the top dogs, I asked myself, *How could this happen? What would the result have been if arsenic erroneously had been used instead? How many people would have died?*

A few years later, I landed the position of Senior Ingredient Buyer, negotiating multi-million dollar contracts for the procurement of the very ingredients that go into our food chain. My days were spent in meetings with the Research and Development teams who tinkered with ingredients and chemicals, trying to attain a product formulation that would be deemed "tasty" in a marketing research panel. Hour upon hour of my time was spent completing detailed business strategies and analyses to determine how much money I could save the company by switching from Ingredient Supplier A to Ingredient Supplier B. I was totally undone when marketing took interest in a cost-savings project that suggested using imitation sugar blueberries in a cereal product to replace the real blueberries that were being used. This little switcheroo would have saved the company two million dollars on an annual basis and my name would have been attached to this foolishness. Thank God, the project was not approved.

After my sixth year in the processed foods industry, I began making a transformation of my own health and eating habits. I had started taking nutritional supplements every day and was making an honest attempt to change my diet by educating myself on the correct foods to eat. I was at peace with eating a salad every day and I had acquired a taste for water instead of sodas. It was not long before I realized there were food products that actually cause more harm to the body than one would expect. Little did I know the contracts I negotiated daily were for the very ingredients used to create these questionable products.

As the buyer for food additives, I became alarmed when I referenced my "food ingredient bible" only to find the artificial colors used to colorize dry drink powders and bottled beverages are derived from coal tar! These very same colors used in food products, pharmaceutical drug tablets, and cosmetics are carcinogenic and are capable of damaging our DNA. Anything that can damage the DNA can harm the immune system, speed up aging, and lead to cancer. No one bothered to tell me this!

I was shocked when I read that chemicals called nitrites, which are used as preservatives in cured meats such as bacon, ham, and lunchmeat to prevent spoilage, actually form cancer-causing compounds known as nitrosamines in the gastrointestinal tract and have been associated with human cancer and birth defects. And here I was supporting one of the top producers of lunchmeat in the world. Weekly, I came across new and mind-boggling information about particular ingredients. My co-workers could not believe it when I shared this information.

Surely, a wholesome company like the one for which I worked would not push products that could potentially cause so much harm, would they? They would if it was profitable and if the workers behind the scenes were uneducated in nutrition! The more and more I learned about nutrition, the more I understood the motives of the industry. In less than a year, I came to understand the processed foods industry was just that — an industry. I faced up to the reality that selling a cheap, nutrition-less product at the lowest price to a large number of repeat consumers makes money.

Like the U.S. healthcare industry, the processed foods industry is a $1 trillion industry. There are just a handful of key players who, through the process of mergers and acquisitions, now control the entire food chain and much of the food choices available to us. My former employers were two of the four major conglomerates. Like athletes at the Olympics, these few companies are all in competition ... competition to launch the most creative, colorful, and sensory-appealing product in the shortest amount of time, in an effort to generate the greatest amount of profit. Nutrition is not the primary objective.

The processed foods market is a land where words such as "innovative," "brand equity," and "convenience" resonate in the hallways. Chemical engineers and food scientists formulate foods in the same way they might formulate laundry detergent. One chemical after another is added to the mix. The product developers receive their direction from marketing MBAs who are paid very comfortable incomes to come up with creative new product ideas. Their crafty marketing techniques are used to get consumers to buy nutrient-deficient, toxin-containing, dead foods.

Economist Paul Zane Pilzner, in his book *The Next Trillion*, sums up the marketing tactics very well.

> In trying to decide what sorts of foods to sell us, they invariably apply one of the great unwritten laws of marketing: It is easier to sell more product to an existing customer than to sell that same product to a new customer. In other words, it is easier to influence a regular customer to eat four additional bags of potato chips per month than it is to persuade a new customer, who may never have tasted potato chips before, to buy even one bag of this new exotic substance. Most processed foods sales, products like Hostess Twinkies, Oreo cookies, and McDonald's Happy Meals, are governed by what those in the business call a "potato chip marketing equation." According to this law, more than 90 percent of product sales are made to less than 10 percent of their customers. In the case of processed foods, that coveted 10 percent consists largely of people weighing more than two hundred pounds earning less than $20,000 per year.

Unless this group of people learns what's really going on, they become locked into this vicious cycle of buying poisonous food year after year.

Within the industry, more emphasis is placed on the packaging of the product than on the product content. The shape. The color pattern. Does it need a flip top? Does it need a no-drip pour spout? Just as Eve was deceived in the garden by her senses, Satan is still using the same old trick. Fancy, brightly-colored packaging is used to lure you in. Children are often the targets as they are attracted to games featured on the packaging or toys buried within. Making food fun is the idea.

Years ago, Kraft's Lunchables won a prize for innovative packaging. However, they bombed in their nutritional scorecard rating. The Center for Science in the Public Interest placed Lunchables on the list of "10 Foods You Should Never Eat!" Its objection to this product is very blunt: "It would be hard to invent a worse food than these combos of heavily processed meat, artery-clogging cheese, and mostly white-flour crackers. The regular lines average four teaspoons of fat and 1,250 mg of sodium. The Deluxe and Fun Packs are even worse. And the Lean Turkey Breast and Cheddar cheese on eight half-dollar sized 'wheat' crackers have as much saturated fat as a couple of pork chops. As for Oscar Mayer's Low Fat and Reduced Fat Lunchables, they may have about half the fat of regular Lunchables, but they are still a junk food." Whew! And you thought you were doing a good thing for your children by sending them off to school with this in their book bags?

You might argue that the processed and fast food companies don't actually *force* people to buy their products. No, they don't. At least not literally. But they do use a tool that has great power of suggestion: television. Food companies know Americans spend an enormous amount of time in front of the television, and as a result, TV commercials are used as an effective means of persuasion. These companies have deep pockets, so the sky is the limit in terms of advertising. In his book *Food Fight*, Kelly D. Brownell, Ph.D., addresses this side of the business: "The advertising budget for soft drinks in 1998 was $115.5 million, for popular candy bars it was $10-$50 million, and for McDonald's the budget was more than $1 billion. Compare that with the National Cancer Institutes' $1 million budget for its 5 A Day campaign or the $1.5 million for the National Cholesterol Education Campaign of the National Heart, Lung, and Blood Institute." Could television be a subtle form of brainwashing? It is if seeing an ad for golden fries prompts you to head for the nearest restaurant drive-through window.

While the industry itself is tainted, the vast majority of people involved in the food production cycle have good intentions. Some honestly believe the work of their hands is producing something convenient enough for a single mother of two to prepare, and colorful enough her children will want to eat it. But dead food is just that. It's worthless because it contains no nutrients. Most processed foods have undergone such extensive manufacturing that the initial food source is no longer recognizable. Rice is heated and puffed to form cereal, and wheat is stripped, ground, heated, molded, and colored to create children's pasta meals. I (Kristy) refer to "dead food" as those food products that do not have significant amounts of vitamins, minerals, fiber, protein, essential fatty acids, and other key components required for life. Rather than being life-enhancing, consumption of these foods can potentially be life-threatening.

The manufactured foods we eat today are vastly different in content from the diets of our ancestors. While they ate fresh home-grown foods, we have resorted to mass-produced items that can be kept for long periods of time before being eaten. Preservatives, including sodium, are added so food items can sit for what seems like an eternity in your kitchen cabinet without growing mold or developing maggots. Ironically, these ingredients are apparently helping another industry save money. I (Kristy) once heard at a health seminar that morticians nowadays are using less embalming fluid on deceased bodies than they did years ago. This is partly due to the fact that bodies are arriving at funeral homes in a pre-preserved state from the chemical food preservatives consumed over the years.

And that's not all. Would you believe some of the materials used to package food products can be dangerous as well? The initial layer of plastic and aluminum packaging takes its toll on the food. From 70 to 80 percent of food is wrapped in various types of plastic, some of which contain potentially cancer-causing agents that migrate into our food.

The chemicals in the plastic liners and containers are just a sample of the 2,500 substances added to the foods we eat during their growth, processing, and packaging; the majority of these substances are toxic to the body. While the body struggles to pass them as waste, many remain behind as accumulative toxins within the cells. Think of toxins as poisonous substances that negatively affect the cells and tissues in the body. Annually, the food industry spends over $4.5 billion on chemical food additives.

Another million-dollar question: Why would anyone want to put chemicals in food? The industry is permitted to do so if the additive: improves the nutritional value (e.g., synthetic vitamins), enhances the quality or consumer acceptability (e.g., artificial flavors and colors), improves the stability, facilitates mass production (e.g., "flow" agents), or makes the food more readily available (e.g., pesticides and herbicides). Again, the industry gets to select which chemicals they can use for their own benefit, yet at our expense.

One such chemical that has been making waves in the industry is diacetyl, which is widely used as a less expensive way to enhance flavor or make food taste like it has butter in it. It is used quite a bit, especially in popcorn. The problem is diacetyl has been linked to a fatal lung disease called "bronchiolitis obliterans." Just in facilities where this chemical is used to flavor popcorn, over two hundred employees have developed lung conditions from bronchiolitis obliterans and at least three people have died from the irreversible disease. An April 2006 Associated Press story reported: "More than 150 former popcorn plant workers have sued companies supplying or making the butter flavoring, and more than $100 million has been awarded in injury verdicts or paid settlement."

Now cases of bronchiolitis obliterans are popping up in other artificial flavoring houses, not just those that make popcorn flavoring. The AP article went on to say, "The Food and Drug Administration (FDA) has allowed flavoring producers and sellers to decide which chemicals are safe, and California's occupational safety agency has delegated health examinations of flavoring workers to an industry-paid doctor." Can you say, "Hush, hush"?

Other chemicals to which we are all probably exposed on a weekly basis are pesticides and fungicides. Did you know 60 percent of all herbicides are carcinogenic, 90 percent of all fungicides are carcinogenic, and 30 percent of all insecticides are carcinogenic? You are probably consuming these harmful agents on your fruits and vegetables. Classified as indirect food additives, nearly one billion pounds of pesticides are applied to crops each year. Allowable residue tolerances are based upon a 160-pound man, yet in 1993 the Environmental Protection Agency (EPA) acknowledged federal safety guidelines for the use of pesticides on food crops should be made ten times more stringent. This acknowledgement was the result of a five-year study of children's health risks commissioned by the National Academy of Sciences (NAS). Their report said children consume higher doses of pesticides than adults due to their body weight. The results often reflect neurological disorders.

With all the chemical warfare taking place in the grocery, is there any hope for consumer protection from these chemicals? Consumer safety is supposed to be guaranteed through a 1958 law called the "Delaney Amendment." This law says food and chemical manufacturers must test additives before they are put on the market, and the tests have to be submitted to the FDA. The law says, "No additive may be permitted in any amount if the tests show it produces cancer when fed to man or animals or by other appropriate tests." Unfortunately, even FDA commissioners claim this law is unenforceable, as they do not have the personnel or resources to prevent all potentially harmful food additives from reaching the market.

According to Ruth Winters, author of *A Consumer's Dictionary of Food Additives*, in 1994 there were 1,149 field officers assigned to consumer safety for the *entire* food, drug, cosmetics, and medical devices categories. Of this number, twenty-nine were toxicologists and twenty were food technologists — obviously not enough staffing to guarantee food safety. In fact, the National Research Council performed an extensive study on food additive testing and toxicity levels in 1980 and anyone would be alarmed by their findings:

- 92 percent of the tests in place were inadequate.
- A large variety of test types were needed, such as chronic studies, inhalation studies, neurotoxicity studies (toxicity to the brain and nerves), genetic toxicity, and effects on the fetus.
- There was no toxicity information available on 46 percent of the additives, and only 5 percent had a complete health-hazard assessment available.

- No toxicity data was available for 80 percent of 49,000 commercially used chemicals.
- Toxicity data was inadequate or nonexistent for 80 percent of 8,600 additives.
- A large percentage of the food additives had not been tested long-term, which is a great problem in determining chemical safety. Cancer, for instance, may take twenty years to develop in humans, and often more than two years to develop in animals. Long-term safety of additives is determined from rats, which only live eighteen to twenty-four months.

The workings of the processed foods industry are aptly described by this passage in Proverbs 14:12: "There is a way which seemeth right unto a man, but the end thereof are the ways of death" (KJV). In an effort to provide the convenience and taste consumers (including church members!) desire, the processed foods industry has neglected to consider a crucial element ... the long-term effects. Their scientific concoctions have been a poor attempt at recreating what God initially put in the Garden of Eden. What God provided to sustain life, man has modified to the point where it can now destroy it.

This chapter would not be complete without introducing you to some of the top ingredients used in the industry. The notoriety of these ingredients stretches beyond the boundaries of the United States, and people around the world are dealing with the consequences of eating foods made from these substances. If ingredients could speak for themselves, they probably would boast about the lives they are destroying. Like the résumé of an honor-roll student, the biographies of these ingredients would be filled with all types of accolades, of which Satan would be proud.

Artificial Flavors

Of all ingredients used in the industry, my family is the largest. I guess we had to be created to replace all the natural flavors lost during the heat-intensive process of manufacturing food. My family tree is vast and our genealogy is about as complicated as that of Abraham, Isaac, Jacob, and Joseph. In my family we have strawberry-banana and banana-strawberry. Grandma always seems to get those two mixed up! A large percentage of my father's side of the family is used extensively in the ice cream industry, otherwise Baskin Robbins would not have achieved its thirty-one flavors. My family is quite popular and I would bet my life there is not one processed food made to which my family and I are not applied. It is said that as much as 50 percent of the hyperactivity in children is caused by my presence.

MSG (Monosodium Glutamate)

I would have to boast I am the granddaddy of all flavoring agents ever created. I pride myself on being the best flavor-enhancer! I am used extensively in the processed food and restaurant industries because when consumed I stimulate the taste cells in the tongue and magnify the flavor of the food. I can make soups and gravies taste better than your grandmother's secret recipes made from scratch. This is why most restaurant meals taste better than foods cooked at home. It's all about me, baby!

Would you believe I make people (young and old) go crazy? Okay, maybe that's an overstatement, but I do have a severe impact on the human mind. Technically classified as an "excitotoxin," I am responsible for several brain disorders such as Parkinson's disease, Huntington's disease, ALS, and Alzheimer's disease. I work best by slowly destroying the brain cells. If I am ingested in large amounts, I can kill off your brain neurons within one hour. Lower doses of me usually take two or more hours to cause the same effect.

No one is exempt from my destruction, not even unborn children. Pregnant women who consume food with me in it increase the child's chances for brain disorders such as autism, learning problems, and hyperactive behavior.

Russell L. Blaylock, M.D., wrote about me in his book, *Excitotoxins: The Taste that Kills.* One passage reads, "Today, virtually all of the neurodegenerative diseases are now considered to be intimately related to the excitotoxic process. Seizures, headaches, strokes, brain injury, subarachnoid hemorrhage, and developmental brain disorders are all intimately related to excitotoxins."

You will find me in canned soup, instant soup, beef or chicken broth, canned food, barbecue sauce, salad dressing, fast food, prepackaged meals, and snack chips to name a few. I am often disguised on ingredient listings as "caseinate," "hydrolyzed vegetable protein," "autolyzed yeast," "yeast extract," "natural flavoring," or "spices." And because the FDA has no restrictions on the amount of MSG that can be added, food processors can go overboard by adding just enough of me to cause you to overeat. "Betcha can't eat just one" takes on a whole new meaning when I'm around.

Sugar

Who am I? Some describe me as likeable but the vast majority of people call me loveable. Many say I am a joy to be around and they could not even think about being without me from morning 'til night. My family is large, and for some reason my parents gave my siblings and me names that seem to rhyme: sucrose, lactose, maltose, dextrose, sucralose, and high fructose corn syrup (that's me). Personally, I consider myself to be a superhero, as there are many feats I can accomplish in just a short period of time. While I won't bore you with all the details, here are just a few:

- I am the primary cause of Type 2 diabetes.
- I am addictive and can be intoxicating, similar to alcohol.
- I have the potential of inducing abnormal metabolic processes in a normal healthy individual and promoting chronic degenerative diseases.
- I can cause arteriosclerosis.
- I can cause cardiovascular disease.
- I can make your skin age by changing the structure of collagen.
- I can cause cataracts.
- I can cause emphysema.
- I can cause free radicals in the blood stream, which can lead to cancer.
- I am a risk factor of gallbladder cancer.
- I increase the risk of gastric cancer.
- I can increase the body's fluid retention.
- I am the number one enemy of the bowel movement, slowing down food's travel time through the gastrointestinal tract.
- I increase the concentration of bile acid in stools and bacterial enzymes in the colon, which can modify bile to produce cancer-causing compounds.
- I cause a depletion in chromium, which is tied to the development and progression of nearsightedness.
- I increase the size of the liver by making the liver cells divide.
- I can increase kidney size and produce pathological changes in the kidney.
- I can damage the pancreas.
- I cause dental cavities.
- I can cause depression.
- I can exacerbate PMS in women.

Artificial Sweeteners (aspartame, saccharin, sucralose)

Those who attempt to make a correction in their diet by first eliminating sugar have no problem finding me. I nest in products labeled as "sugar-free," "diet," and "low-calorie." Hiding out in simple things like chewing gum and toothpaste, I have been known to trick the most die-hard calorie-counter. My success lies in the fact that most people have not learned to look for me in the ingredient listings of food products, but rather they waste their time glaring at the nutritional panel hoping they can make some sense of the limited information provided. I am a trickster ... yes, that old Jacob in the bible had nothing on me.

I am crafty in that I go by many different names. Sometimes I go by "saccharin," sometimes I use my nickname "Sweet'N Low." When I am feeling quite sweet, I like to dress in a little pink package. When dressed in pink, I have been known to cause cancer. Luckily, my designer label on my clothes does not come with a cancer warning, otherwise those who consume me daily in their morning cups of coffee would not care for me as much.

On days when I am feeling kind of blue, I put on my blue outfit and request my friends call me "aspartame," or "Equal" for short. I guess the color blue reflects innocence, kind of like a little baby boy, but my motives are anything but innocent. At 180 times sweeter than sugar and with zero calories, I am now used in over nine thousand consumable food products yielding $1 billion in sales a year. Some would say I am priceless.

A company called Searle initially birthed me to be used as a drug. However, if I had remained classified as a drug, by law my adverse reactions would have to have been reported to consumers. Thank goodness a company called Monsanto adopted me and won my approval with the FDA without having to test me on human beings. Therefore, Monsanto earned the license to market me as a food additive rather than a drug, and I received free reign to create havoc in the lives of many.

I am responsible for 75 percent of all adverse reactions reported to the FDA. A few feats of which I am quite proud include: initiation or aggravation of diabetes mellitus, hypoglycemia, convulsions, headache, depression and other irregular psychiatric states, hyperthyroidism, hypertension, arthritis, the simulation of multiple sclerosis, Alzheimer's disease, lupus, addiction, brain tumors, pseudotumor (a neurological condition in overweight young women), and carpal tunnel syndrome.

Currently, a major food manufacturer is working day and night to further promote my presence in ethnic neighborhoods where diabetes is a common killer. Unfortunately, consumers are not being clued in to the warning label that comes on my blue outfit, as well as on any food package that contains me. "Phenylketonurics," it says, always written in bold black or red lettering. When consumers begin to develop headaches, which can lead to seizures in some cases, they have no idea the phenylketonurics label was a warning sign that their brain cells are being destroyed with no room for reversal.

My favorite days are when the sun shines. The sun just makes me feel splendid, so I put on my yellow outfit and go by the name "sucralose," a.k.a. "Splenda." Folks don't know that in order to make me, regular sugar molecules are tainted with toxic chlorine molecules. That's right! Good old chlorine — the same stuff used to clean swimming pools. I am six hundred times sweeter than regular sugar and am touted as the best stuff since sliced bread because I have zero calories. However, new research is indicating long-term health problems could result from my consumption.

Confession of a Soft Drink (author unknown)

Hello. I am a humble, effervescent liquid. Humble? Well, that is debatable. Actually, I am quite proud of myself. Allow me to brag a little.

I fizz, sparkle, and bubble my way into thousands of people all over the world every day. I have much power! I can cause masses of humanity to rush to snack dispensers in plush high-rise buildings. I stir men, women, and teenagers to dash into their cars late at night and speed to their nearest twenty-four-hour convenience stores. I motivate others to root through their purses for their last pennies, nickels, dimes, and quarters with which they will gladly part in exchange for me. The best thing about me is: I am habit forming. I am responsible for giving thousands of addicts their daily fixes. This is because I sometimes contain a substance called "caffeine."

Caffeine is a stimulant. And when people consume drinks with caffeine, it makes their hearts beat very fast and their nervous systems work like crazy. They feel as though they could take on the world. I tell you, I have overwhelming personal magnetism. I'm a sneaky double agent, too. I pretend to give people all the good they need because caffeine gives them a "lift." However, a few hours afterward, they come crashing down, get shaky, and need me again for another pseudo-charge. This plays havoc with their hearts and nerves, but they still look to me for relief. I feel very, very smug because I call the shots!

To give me an appetizing brown tint, I contain "caramel coloring," which has genetic effects and is a cancer-causing suspect. I sometimes have polyethylene glycol as one of my ingredients. Glycol is used as anti-freeze in automobiles and as an oil solvent.

The bubbles and fizz, which potently burn human insides, are caused by my phosphoric acid and carbon dioxide. The phosphorus in the acid upsets the body's calcium-phosphorus ratio and dissolves calcium out of the bones. This can eventually result in osteoporosis, a weakening of the skeletal structure, which can make a person susceptible to broken bones. Also, the phosphorus fights with the hydrochloric acid in human stomachs and renders it ineffective. This promotes indigestion, bloating, and gassiness in many individuals. Carbon dioxide is a waste product exhaled by humans, but they ingest it when they drink me. Some might think I should be more humble about my abilities. But why should I be? Look what I can do!

Salt

Hey, there! You may call me "salt," but my real name is "sodium chloride." I, too, am a chemically processed substance. My twin brother, sea salt, is far superior and healthier than I, but many mistake me for him anyway and assume there is no difference between us. I am used in the majority of processed foods because I am good at killing bacteria. In fact, I have a Master of Science degree in B.K. (bacteria killing). Food manufacturers and retailers love me because I also kill the life force in food, which is a key secret to keeping food on a grocery shelf for months or in a can for years. In human beings, I go directly for the cardiovascular system. If I can get you to consume me in excess through bags of chips and saltines, then I can provoke a potassium deficiency that will shrink, calcify, scar, and destroy the muscles, valves, and arteries along your entire coronary route, with congestive heart failure as a realistic possibility.

Partially Hydrogenated Oils (Trans Fats)

If you are munching on snack food products such as chips and microwave popcorn, then you are most likely consuming me. However, some manufacturers say they are giving me the boot, thanks to pressure from the "good health" police. I am produced when hydrogen gas is added under extreme pressure to liquid oil, the purpose of which is to convert liquid oils to semi-solid fats at room temperature. If you have ever seen the contents of a can of Crisco, then you have seen me. Some say I have a strong resemblance to plastic inside the body. Used extensively in the food and restaurant industries, my purpose is to provide an inexpensive way for manufacturers to keep their products fresher longer.

Because I am cheap and shelf-stable, I have replaced lard in fast-food restaurant baking and frying. Not only am I capable of increasing your bad cholesterol (LDL), I pride myself on also lowering your good cholesterol (HDL). I guess you could say I am an instigator of heart disease.

Despite my history, people still can't stop consuming me. That's because they find products made with me, such as pre-packaged cakes, pies, doughnuts, and cookies, far too irresistible. I put the filling in Twinkies and other snack cakes. Even diners in restaurants compliment the results of my presence in fried foods such as French fries, onion rings, mozzarella sticks, and chicken wings. You can thank me for the three sticks of margarine your mom might put in your favorite cake. For the life of me, I can't figure out why anyone would choose me over butter but I'm so glad so many people do!

In his book *Beating the Food Giants*, Paul A Stitt gave reference to me by saying, "Harvard School of Public Health published in a prestigious British medical journal that four servings of white bread, cake, or cookies that contain partially hydrogenated fats can increase the chances of heart trouble by 67 percent, or two-and-a-half pats of margarine can increase the chance of heart trouble by 100 percent." Perhaps when enough people fall dead while spreading me on their toast, they will better understand I was never meant to be consumed and leave me alone. Meanwhile, I just love being so popular!

Enriched White Flour

Americans love me! They consume me at least three times a day. In the morning, I am found in their bagels, muffins, Pop-Tarts, and pancakes. At lunchtime, I am the foundation for their Subway sandwich or their five-topping pizza. Then at dinnertime, I make up their entire meal of lasagna and garlic bread. "The whiter the bread, the quicker the dead" is what I often chant. I contain absolutely no nutritional value. Because of how the wheat used to make me is milled, 90 percent of my nutrients are removed and fed to cattle. I guess that is why the word "enriched" has to be added to the packages of bread products made with me. This way, the consumer sees the iron and other vitamins and minerals used for chemical enrichment, although these nutrients are not fully absorbable by the body.

So I may appear white as snow, I have to undergo a bleaching process. Unfortunately, one of the chemicals that may be used — chlorine dioxide — is toxic to the body. Do you remember when you were in elementary school and made paste from water and flour in order to complete your papier mâché project? I was the one who got stirred up in the water. If I could make paste back then, I am still capable of making paste today — but in your digestive system. Please give me all the credit for your weekly bouts of constipation.

Do you feel well acquainted with these ingredients now? In their infinite wisdom, the corporate giants and creative technologists feel they can continue to develop cheap, imitation food and market it as being wholesome. The principle of man-made food is against the will of our Father. When the Israelites left Egypt, they survived on a daily supply of manna. Manna, the Hebrew name given to this daily bread, means "What is it"? This unknown substance came directly from heaven, with no extended shelf life.

> *And when the dew had gone, behold, upon the face of the wilderness there lay a fine, round flakelike thing, as fine as hoarfrost on the ground. When the Israelites saw it, they said one to another, Manna [What is it?]. For they did not know what it was. And Moses said to them, "This is the bread which the Lord has given you to eat". This is what the Lord has commanded: Let every man gather of it as much as he will need, an omer for each person, according to the number of your persons: take it, every man for those in his tent. The [people] did so, and gathered, some more, some less. When they measured it with an omer, he who gathered much had nothing over, and he who gathered little had no lack; each gathered according to his need. Moses said, Let none of it be left until morning. But they did not listen to Moses; some of them left of it until morning, and it bread worms, became foul, and stank; and Moses was angry with them. ~ Exodus 16:14-20 (AMP)*

The manna was a complete, wholesome food that met all of the children of Israel's nutritional needs for forty years; it was divine health food. It rained down fresh every day. It could not be preserved. When a few of the Israelites attempted to store away some of the manna to eat later, it spoiled and smelled badly.

Think about it. If fresh bread is left unattended on a kitchen counter for a few days, it should spoil and start growing mold. I challenge you to put a loaf of your favorite white bread on the table for a week and observe what happens ... absolutely nothing! The bread does not spoil because during the wheat production process, the most nutritious sections of the wheat kernel — which are also the parts that spoil very easily — are removed. For this reason, white flour is void of key nutrients and is lacking in fiber. The end result is a toxic paste that contributes heavily to constipation and colon cancer. Now suppose what would have happened if Wonder Bread had fallen from the sky instead of manna? The children of

Israel might not have ever made it into Canaan. If they had, they might have been quite feeble and sickly, a stark contrast to the good health they had when they originally left Egypt.

As I (Kristy) frequently share these facts and figures on processed foods during my nutritional seminars and workshops, the attendees all respond in the same manner. Their mouths are left hanging wide open, speechless about our nation's food chain. Many shake their heads in disbelief and some even get angry and defiant. Taking all responses into consideration, the overall theme is universal. Most walk away saying, "We didn't know." At one point in time, I, too, was unaware. I praise God he chose me to be his agent behind the scenes so the truth could be brought to you. I have seen far too many people being destroyed for a lack of knowledge (Hosea 4:6). Don't stay in the dark with them.

Chapter Summary

1. Satan is using specific food ingredients as weapons against you.
2. Just because a food or a food ingredient has been approved for use does not always mean it is safe to consume.
3. Key ingredients to look for and avoid in product ingredient listings include:
   a. Artificial colors
   b. Nitrates
   c. Artificial flavors
   d. MSG (monosodium glutamate)
   e. Sugar
   f. Sugar substitutes: aspartame (Equal), saccharin (Sweet'N Low), sucralose (Splenda)
   g. Soda/Caffeine
   h. Salt
   i. Partially hydrogenated oils (trans fats)
   j. Enriched white flour

Chapter Fourteen

Casualties of War

But your little ones, whom you said would be victims, I will bring in, and they shall know the land which you have despised. ~ Numbers 14:31

Scene 1: Mrs. Johnson's Second Grade Classroom

Seven-year-old Jake is not paying attention. His tummy is churning. The sausage and cheese biscuit he ate for breakfast is about to reappear. Little Amy has asthma and feels an attack coming on and is feverishly searching for her inhaler. Thomas was diagnosed in first grade with ADHD (Attention Deficit Hyperactivity Disorder). Because he did not take his Ritalin this morning, it is impossible for him to sit still in his seat. Belinda is overweight and is sitting by herself because the other children always make fun of her. They call her "Big Butt Belinda." Out of twenty-eight students, eight are out sick with the flu and another five are wheezing, coughing, and wiping their runny noses. The eight who are absent have been out for over a week and will have a hard time catching up on their schoolwork after they return.

Scene 2: The School Cafeteria

The lunch line is long today because the most-favored fare, pizza and French fries, is being served, albeit for the third time this week. The kids jokingly call the pizza "government cheese on cardboard," but they go for it every time it's on the menu. Their number two favorite — French fries — are dripping with grease. The snack bar is full of activity. Kids line up for chips, ice cream, candy bars, doughnuts, and other cream-filled pastries. Susie has given her best friend Katie a dollar to buy a soda from one of the seven vending machines in the cafeteria. Betsy's mom packed her lunch and included an apple and carrot sticks. Betsy is trying to trade them for a sticky bun. There are no takers.

Scene 3: After School

Aaron went to his friend Tony's house after school. Tony's parents weren't home. The two boys played video games, joked about skipping gym class, ate chilidogs and tortilla chips, and drank orange soda. Tony's mom had baked a carrot cake the day before, so the boys helped themselves to huge slices. When Aaron returned home, he took his insulin right on schedule.

Scene 4: Dinner at Home

It's dinner at Shanna's house. Her mom made Hamburger Helper and canned green beans. Shanna hates Hamburger Helper so she toyed with her food a bit before excusing herself from the table. She said she had had a big lunch and wasn't very hungry. After her mom went to bed, Shanna microwaved the Taco Bell burrito she had stashed away in the refrigerator two days before. She washed it down with Sunny Delight, grabbed some M&M's, and went to bed. At two a.m., she woke up her mom and asked for Alka-Seltzer.

These are just hypotheticals, yet they are not out of the ordinary in homes and schools across America. It is all too easy to substitute the names of children we know into these scenarios. Your daughter, Alyssa; your neighbor's son, Calvin; your niece, Stephanie; your grandson, David. The names change but the impact is the same for all of these little ones. In sum, more and more American children are setting themselves up for destruction. They are eating themselves to death, just like some of their parents.

Among children and teens ages six to nineteen, 16 percent (over nine million) are overweight. This figure is triple the percentage of overweight children in 1980. Statistics from the American Obesity Association show the prevalence of obesity quadrupled over the past twenty-five years for young boys and girls, as well as doubled over the past twenty-five years for adolescents. In December 2006, the *American Journal of Public Health* published a study that said over a third of three-year-olds from low-income families in twenty major cities are overweight or obese. Ethnically, the numbers break down this way: 32 percent white, 32 percent black, and 44 percent Hispanic.

The number of health problems children face has risen right along with their weight. According to a National Health and Nutrition Examination Survey, hypertension among American children and teenagers has steadily increased over the last decade. The disease is common among African-American and Hispanic children. It gets worse. An estimated 10 percent of all children have cholesterol levels above the recommended range, making them susceptible to heart disease as adults. Diseases that at one time only showed up in adults and took thirty to forty years to develop are now being diagnosed in children as young as five or six. In *Food Fight*, author Kelly Brownell says, "Type 2 (adult-onset diabetes) is starting to occur in children. Children who develop Type 2 diabetes may have heart attacks and need coronary bypass surgery before they reach age 30."

These statistics are alarming! How is it that innocent children, whose lives consist of nothing more than eating, going to school, playing, watching television, and sleeping, could be set up for such failure? What kind of future can any child born in the United States expect to have, given these devastating numbers?

To find solutions and possibly provide an ounce of hope for Generations Y and Z, parents must look for areas in our culture that drive these results — places where lifestyle defenses are weak and dietary attacks are more likely to occur. School is a no-brainer. Officials are on heightened alert when it comes to protecting students from school shootings and other random violence. But the attacks they face between eleven a.m. and one p.m. are largely ignored. Instead of filling up at lunchtime on nutritious fuel, children have the chance to eat a bunch of junk that sends them on a "sugar high." Wiped out by the white stuff, they typically have a less productive afternoon back in the classroom. You might say vending machines and other lunchroom menu items victimize them.

Food industry lobbyists have created mandatory school lunch and milk programs consisting of processed foods that can become addictive. I (Kristy) challenge you to go into any school cafeteria and look at what is being served. You'll find the staple is a hamburger and French fries, followed by a sugar-filled dessert. Very few *real* fruits and vegetables are on site, and if they are, many children are apparently not eating them.

Over 99,000 public and private schools participate in the National School Lunch Program (NSLP), which offers low-cost or sometimes even free lunches; however, even a federally funded program such as this has its flaws. Author Brownell says, "Many of the foods offered through this program are animal products rich in cholesterol and saturated fat — the same type of fat the United Stated Department of Agriculture (USDA) recommends schools reduce. Even when schools do attempt to order the more nutritious items from commodity lists, they are often unable to do so due to low demand from other schools and, therefore, infrequent delivery of these items."

In order to satisfy a child's protein needs, a carton of cow's milk is always provided as part of the NSLP. More so, television commercials suggest that everyone should consume dairy products such as milk, cheese, yogurt, and ice cream because, not only do they taste good, but they appear to "do a body good" as well. If we were alive during the biblical era, there may be some merit found in this media message. However, today's research suggests otherwise.

Let's start from the beginning – where does milk come from and what is its purpose? All mammals (humans and some animal species) produce milk for the sole purpose of providing nourishment and transporting hormones from mother to child. For an infant, breast milk truly is the ultimate superfood! It contains a perfect nutrient balance of protein, fat, and carbohydrates necessary to meet the needs of a growing infant. The large percentage of fat and cholesterol are essential for the growth and development of the infant's brain and for proper absorption of minerals and the fat-soluble vitamins D, E, A, and K. Digestive enzymes such as lipase for breaking down fat, and lactase for breaking down the lactose (milk sugar) are also available in breast milk.

Nowadays, many women are choosing man-made formula over the powerful properties of breast milk, and ultimately, their children are suffering. Studies of children from infancy to age five, whereby they were breast-fed, have shown that these children have a much lower incidence of diarrhea, urinary tract infections, pneumonia, vomiting, asthma, earaches, childhood allergies, bacterial infections, cancers, and learning disabilities. This is in part due to the abundance of colostrum that is passed from mother to child during breast-feeding. Colostrum is a nutrient that is instrumental in building the child's immune system.

So, it is apparent that breast milk is the ideal food for infants, but should we be drinking pasteurized cow milk and eating dairy-based products once weaned? To find our answer, we must go to the source – the Bible. The Bible does clearly indicate that milk from cows, goats, sheep, and camels was consumed during biblical times. Obviously, there weren't any refrigerators back then and milk could not be stored. Instead, it was fermented to keep it from spoiling. Cheese, butter, and yogurt (sour milk) were available as a result of fermentation.

And he took butter, and milk, and the calf which he had dressed, and set it before them; and he stood by them under the tree, and they did eat. ~ Genesis 18:8 (KJV)

And thou shalt have goats' milk enough for thy food, for the food of thy household, and for the maintenance for thy maidens. ~ Proverbs 27:27 (KJV)

*Butter of kine, and milk of sheep, with fat of lambs, and rams of
the breed of Bashan, and goats, with the fat of kidneys of wheat;
and thou didst drink the pure blood of the grape.*
~ *Deuteronomy 32:14 (KJV)*

*Thirty milk camels with their colts, 40 cows, 10 bulls, 20 she-
donkeys, and 10 (donkey) colts.* ~ *Genesis 32:15 (AMP)*

Surely the churning of milk bringeth forth butter.
~ *Proverbs 30:33 (KJV)*

Ideally, if milk was good for Abraham, Isaac, Joseph, and Jesus, then it could be deduced that it could be beneficial for you and me. This would be a true statement if man had not started tinkering around with milk. Selective breeding, as well as the handling of dairy products has changed extensively in the past 2,000 years, which has made milk lose its "good health status" and instead has placed milk on the list of the top ten foods to avoid. Frankly, neither children nor adults should consume the pasteurized dairy products that are now sold in U.S. groceries.

To understand why modern milk is harmful, you must look at its components. Milk from cattle (bovine milk) is made up of water, fats, protein, minerals, and lactose (milk sugar). It is the protein component that is of key concern and can be problematic. There are two types of milk protein – casein which is in solid form, and whey which is in liquid form. While all milk contains both types of protein, the milk from "black and white" cows of American and European descent (USA, Canada, Britain, and much of Scandinavia) carry a unique protein called A1 beta-casein protein. A1 beta-casein milk, which is what you will find in most U.S. stores, has been implicated in Type I diabetes, autism, heart disease, leaky gut syndrome, milk allergies, excess mucous production, and a host of auto-immune conditions.

According to the American Academy of Allergy, Asthma, and Immunology, cow's milk is the number one cause of food allergies in children. The *American Journal of Nutrition* says, "A study of children in forty countries found the incidence of juvenile diabetes was directly related to diet. The higher the consumption of cow's milk and other animal products, the greater the chance of developing diabetes." In another study of eight hundred children, researchers found giving them cow's milk products before age eight created a risk factor for juvenile diabetes, and that breast-feeding babies for more than the first week after birth protected infants from developing diabetes (Diabetes Care, Gimeno et al., August 1997).

It is important to note that milk from Asian and African breeds of cows, as well as goats' milk and human milk, are free from the A1 beta-casein, which is the basis for the aforementioned studies. Asian and African cows contain what is called A2 beta-casein which is acceptable by the body and does not pose health challenges. Ironically, all milk (including "biblical milk") used to be A2 classified milk until a natural mutation affected some European cows a long time ago. Today, healthy "A2 milk" sourced from Asian and African cows is available in countries such as New Zealand. You can wager that due to economic reasons, the breeding of A2 cows and the commercialization of dairy products derived from A2 milk is still being kept a big secret here in the U.S. To divulge such a secret could potentially upset our dairy and medical/insurance industries, and why would we do that? Imagine the financial ripple effect that might occur should the USDA finally admit that U.S. dairy is responsible for sickness. We might see quite a bit of milk, cheese and ice cream spoiling in grocery stores nationwide and an industry counting huge economic losses if consumers are put on notice. As they wean themselves from dairy and its associated side effects, their doctor visits might decrease. Consequently, the physician's income as well as the insurance industry's profit margin might see a reduction.

This history of modern milk gets worse…

In 1920, pasteurization of milk was introduced merely to kill the bacteria in milk. Once outlawed for health reasons, pasteurization became the standard practice due to political lobbying. Pasteurization involves heating the milk to 160 degrees for 45 minutes in an effort to kill bacteria. This process is done now primarily to extend the shelf-life of milk. Thus, we can conveniently store milk in our refrigerators for over a week, as opposed to going out and milking a cow as was done in the good old days. While pasteurization may zap out the bad bugs, it also destroys a good amount of key nutrients found in milk, including vitamin C, enzymes, amino acids, fatty acids, and vitamins A, C, and D. Fifty percent of the calcium and magnesium are lost during pasteurization, not to mention that these minerals require enzymes in order for the body to absorb them.

And if pasteurization is not bad enough, the milk makers now homogenize milk. Homogenization breaks up the larger fat molecules in whole milk into very tiny molecules, which suspends them evenly in milk. This creates a very smooth, consistent milk that does not require stirring when it is stored. While this process seems ideal, it makes milk a prime suspect in heart disease. Why? When milk is not homogenized, the large fat molecules are able to pass through the intestines. However, the tiny fat molecules of homogenized milk tend to pass through the intestinal wall and into the bloodstream. The result is an increase in our triglyceride and cholesterol levels. Additionally, an enzyme found in the homogenized milk fat – xanthine oxidase –

further damages the smooth lining of blood vessels, contributing to buildup of plaque in the arteries.

A subtle fear exists around the notion that raw, non-pasteurized dairy products cause heart disease in the same manner as pasteurized, homogenized dairy products. Sally Fallon and Mary Enig, Ph.D., clear up this fatty subject in the book *Nourishing Traditions: The Cookbook that Challenges Politically Correct Nutrition and the Diet Dictocrats* by stating:

> The cause of heart disease is not animal fats and cholesterol but rather a number of factors inherent in modern diets, including excess consumption of vegetable oils and hydrogenated fats; excess consumption of refined carbohydrates in the form sugar and white flour; mineral deficiencies; particularly low levels of protective magnesium and iodine; deficiencies of vitamins, particularly vitamin C, needed for integrity of the blood vessel walls, and of antioxidants like selenium and vitamin E, which protect us from free radicals; and finally the disappearance of antimicrobial fats from the food supply, namely animal fats and tropical oils.

What's the final verdict on the bright, white stuff? It can be acceptable to consume dairy products today as long as they are derived from healthy, organic, hormone-free, A2-classified cows, and are low-heat processed (non-pasteurized and non-homogenized). You may have to do a bit of hunting to find them, but they are out there. One such reputable company, *Beyond Organic*, offers such cultured dairy products including yogurt and cheese.

While schools play a fundamental role in the development and education of children, they are not always funded appropriately. To make up for the money shortage, schools unfortunately have turned to soft drink and snack food manufacturers for help. Vending machines are seen as the ultimate financial solution because schools receive compensation from product sales. The result is vending machines in schools that carry, soda, candy bars, snack chips, pretzels, etc. Too bad the items in the vending machines don't come with plain and simple written warnings that say, "Stop! I contain products that can harm you!" Believe it or not, vending machines are a common sight in schools from elementary to high school, and have proven to be quite lucrative. "Schools receive only $2.14 for each free meal they serve as part of the National School Lunch Program, often not enough to break even, but the profit margins on a la carte foods and items sold in vending machines can be 50 percent to 100 percent," says Brownell in *Food Fight*.

With all the sugar and grease children are allowed to consume each day, teachers should not be surprised as to why little Thomas cannot pay attention in class and spends his time talking and bothering his classmates. Many times the school system will rush to slap the ADD/ADHD label upon Thomas's forehead. According to the *Diagnostic and Statistical Manual of Mental Disorders,* published by the American Psychiatric Association, a child may be diagnosed with ADHD if he or she shows a disturbance of at least six months during which at least eight of the following are present in the child:

1. Often fidgets with hands or feet and squirms in seat
2. Has difficulty remaining seated when required to do so
3. Is easily distracted
4. Has difficulty awaiting turn in games or group situations
5. Often blurts out answers to questions before they have been completed
6. Has difficulty following through on instructions from others
7. Has difficulty sustaining attention in tasks or play activities
8. Often shifts from one uncompleted activity to another
9. Has difficulty playing quietly
10. Often talks excessively
11. Often interrupts or intrudes on others; example: butts into other children's games
12. Often does not seem to listen to what is being said to him or her
13. Often loses things necessary for tasks or activities at school or at home; examples: toys, pencils, books, assignments
14. Often engages in physically dangerous activities without considering the possible consequences; example: runs into the street without looking

Because there is not presently an independent test that can medically determine if a child has ADHD, these subjective tests and assessments by adults can possibly ruin a child for life. Interesting, huh? Children who could possibly be demonstrating the effects of nutritional deficiencies (hyperactivity, lack of focus, disruptive behavior) are penalized for expressing a natural biological reaction.

In America alone, 2.5 million children have been labeled with ADHD and 4 to 12 percent of six- to twelve-year-olds have been diagnosed with ADD/ADHD. For treatment, these children are given stimulant drugs such as Ritalin, Adderall, Strattera, and Concerta. In fact, between 1999 and 2003, 78 million prescriptions were written for

ADHD drugs in children. (Well Being Journal, Volume 16, No. 2 March/April 2007 and "Drugging Our Children – the Physical, Emotional and Psycho-social Impact of Psychotropic Drugs on the Development of Children", by Gwen Olsen).

Every day, around six million children, some as young as two or three, are given Ritalin at the urging of school officials and psychiatrists. What parents don't realize is use of Ritalin is much more serious than they may have been told. "Drugging Our Children," an article in the March/April 2007 issue of *Well Being Journal*, reports, "In 1971, the Drug Enforcement Administration classified Ritalin (methylphenidate) along with other amphetamine drugs as Schedule II substances, based on the United Nations Convention on Psychotropic Substances. This category indicates these drugs have significant risk of abuse and limited medicinal value. Other Schedule II drugs include: cocaine, morphine, opium, and barbiturates."

Ritalin affects the body both chemically and neurologically. It overwhelms the child's central nervous system and cuts the child's motors, causing the child to go into a state of stupor. The result is a child appears quieter and less active. What is the long-term result of continued use? The longer a child is on Ritalin, the greater the potential consequences.

A recent review conducted by the FDA found almost 1,000 reports of psychosis or mania possibly linked to ADHD drugs — which included Adderall, Concerta, Ritalin, and Strattera — from Jan. 1, 2000 through June 30, 2005. A large number of the psychosis-related cases were reported in children ten years of age or less, an age group not highly predisposed to psychotic episodes. Many suffered from both visual and tactile hallucinations involving insects, snakes, and worms. The FDA estimates that only one to ten percent of all adverse reactions are identified and reported. Because of their unique biological makeup and developing kidneys and livers, it is often difficult for children to metabolize and eliminate drugs, or they can be rapid metabolizers and experience withdrawal between doses. They are three times as likely as adults to experience adverse pharmacologic reactions and interactions.

~ "Drugging Our Children," *Well Being Journal*, March/April 2007

And if adverse reactions to the drug are not enough to worry about, add destructive or harmful behavior to your list of concerns. Forty-six percent of children on Ritalin are charged with at least one major felony by age eighteen and suicide is a common "symptom" of withdrawal from this dangerous drug. The causes are obvious and the solutions are simple. Children are not born Ritalin deficient, they merely become deficient of key nutrients required to support proper brain function, which is crucial in preventing ADHD. "Whole Food Nutrition," an article in the March/April 2007 issue of *Well Being Journal*, reported, "In addition to EFA deficiencies (essential fatty acids, or good fats), numerous studies have indicated specific vitamin and mineral deficiencies in ADHD sufferers." Some of these vital nutrients include zinc, which is found in whole grains, and magnesium, which is found in dark green vegetables — two food groups to which most children are not routinely exposed.

Even if your child's health is not ruined at school, he or she could run a risk of damage at home. Check your kitchen cupboards. Check your refrigerator. Read the labels. If you cannot pronounce an ingredient listed on a package, it could be a bullet aimed at your family's vital organs. Sure it will take a while to penetrate, but it might eventually destroy their health. Your kids learn by watching you.

Patterns of eating microwaveable pastries for breakfast, stuffed pizza for lunch, and fast food for dinner can become engraved in stone in your child's mind. Breakfast should be one of the most important and healthiest meals of the day. But, some parents succumb to convenience by offering their children frozen waffles easily heated in a toaster before being draped with high fructose corn syrup. If frozen delicacies are not provided, then sugary, glazed pastries are served. "Dunkin' Donuts sells 6.4 million donuts per day (enough to circle the earth twice), totaling 2.3 billion donuts per year," says Brownell in *Food Fight*. Children can just grab these tasty little round pastries and eat on the go since no cooking is required. But this easy snack can also be an easy way to a heart attack down the road.

For in between meals, chips, peanut butter, and cheese and crackers are standard menu options. And if a child is thirsty, artificially colored sugar-water is provided in a creative container that allows a child to have fun while sipping. Today's children are enticed into wanting these creative items through the same medium that influences adult lifestyles: the television. Usually, in an effort to delay starting their homework, children will spend a few hours plopped in front of the TV as soon as they get home from school. Brownell says in *Food Fight*, "About $10 billion per year is spent on advertising food to children. Children see ten advertisements per hour when they watch TV, most of them for unhealthy foods." In fact, half of all ads shown during Saturday morning shows are for food, primarily targeted at children.

The persuasive tools of advertising – flavor, color, magic, and convenience are in effect destroying the eating habits of both children and their parents. Research has shown that children's poor eating habits can be linked to the amount of television they watch. As children learn of a new, innovative snack food that has hit the scene, they exercise their buying power by influencing their parents to purchase the item. The bottom line is, when it comes to nutrition, as well as electronics and cars, children are not qualified to make decisions. "A study of children ages six through eight found 70 percent believed fast foods were healthier than food from the home. A study of Australian children ages nine to ten indicated more than half believe Ronald McDonald knows best what children should eat" says Brownell in *Food Fight*. Again, children should not serve as guides; they need to be guided.

Even if you health-proof your home and control what your child eats at school, there is always the mall. This popular kid hangout is full of potentially lethal meals. And food courts offer just about any kind of poison they want. These places seduce your kids with clever marketing and low costs. Satan charges little for the bullets that inflict the wounds, but will try to take every dime we have to remedy the condition. Allergies. Diabetes. Obesity. The conditions seem to grow worse and our children expand wider.

The origins of childhood obesity can be linked to the dramatic shift in the labor market over the last thirty years. As the U.S. workforce has developed into a two-income market whereby both parents are now forced to work in order to make ends meet, less time is allotted to cooking well-balanced nutritious meals. A lifestyle of eating fast food and preservative-laden microwave meals, often late at night, has been adopted.

Children who have less parental supervision often are left making decisions in the kitchen that really should be made by adults. But whose responsibility is it to protect them and ensure their health is maintained and sickness and disease are avoided? Is it their teacher's job? Should Mrs. Johnson be held accountable if little Betsy trades her apple packed in her school lunch for a sticky bun? Is it their doctor's responsibility? Absolutely not! Disease prevention must begin at home. It is the parents' responsibility to ensure their children receive the proper nourishment, both at home and away from home.

In essence, children must be trained in every area of their lives, including dietary habits. Proverbs 22:6 says, "Train up a child in the way he should go, and when he is old, he will not depart from it." So, if a child is taught healthy eating habits early on, he or she will more likely keep them through adulthood. It has been said a child begins to identify his likes and dislikes regarding food around age three. By the time a child is eight years old, his or her eating habits are pretty much established for life.

Imagine what would happen if a young child were raised in a household where the kitchen was seldom used and fast food was a way of life. This child would have absolutely no knowledge of or desire to eat healthy items such as fruit and vegetables. As a result, his poor eating early on in life would paint a bleak picture of his state of health later on down the road. Unfortunately, the future does not look good. American children may be the first generation in history to live shorter lives than their parents did. Neglecting to train up a child in the area of healthy eating contributes to the problem.

God's desire for parents to train up their children is all for one reason: protection. He loves us so much that he has his eyes (not to mention the eyes of his many angels) upon us at all times for our protection. Like a precious artifact, we are God's creation, and he desires to preserve that which he has created. "The Lord shall preserve you from all evil; he shall preserve your soul. The Lord shall preserve your going out and your coming in from this time forth, and even evermore" (Psalm 121:7-8).

At a very young age, children are taught by their parents not to play in the street. Upon seeing a child wander aimlessly into oncoming traffic, parents will risk their own lives in an effort to protect that precious seed. You bundle up your child when it's cold outside. You carefully screen his or her friends and the TV shows they watch — or at least you should. Many parents monitor kids' Internet activities. But how are you protecting your young one in the midst of the current health crisis? How would you rate yourself on safeguarding your children's health?

Psalm 127:3 says, "Behold, children are a heritage from the Lord, the fruit of the womb is a reward." Children are a blessing and a reward from above and God wants to protect this precious seed. The seed is an important element in the Bible.

And God said, Let the earth put forth [tender] vegetation: plants yielding seed and fruit trees yielding fruit whose seed is in itself, each according to its kind, upon the earth. And it was so. The earth brought forth vegetation: plants yielding seed according to their own kinds and trees bearing fruit in which was their seed, each according to its kind. And God saw that it was good [suitable, admirable] and He approved it. ~ Genesis 1:11-12 (AMP)

This concept of multiplication and duplication was carried beyond the scope of plant vegetation with the creation of Adam and Eve. Adam and Eve were God's first seed upon the earth. As the seed of a plant carries all the pertinent genes to duplicate that particular plant species, Adam and Eve were created with divine DNA to be just like God. They were made in his image and in his likeness. And in Genesis 1:28, God gives this couple instructions for starting the first heavenly family on earth: "Be fruitful and multiply; fill the earth." Because Adam and Eve were connected and abiding continually with God, they had his protection twenty-four hours a day.

There are several incidents where God goes out of his way to protect and preserve the seed. In Genesis, when Eve said the serpent, which was merely the seed of Satan, coerced her into taking a bite of the forbidden fruit, God immediately put into action a plan whereby the product of a "seed" would be the ultimate hero for mankind. He spoke directly to the serpent with his foolproof plan, which was far too complex for Satan to comprehend: "And I will put enmity between you and the woman, and between your seed and her Seed; he shall bruise your head, and you shall bruise His heel" (Genesis 3:15). Stated in "code," this was God's plan for the redemption of man, or the future offspring of Adam and Eve. It would be the seed of a woman that would play a critical role in undoing the mistake of Adam and Eve in the garden. That seed is none other than Jesus Christ.

After Adam's death, and as people began to multiply on the face of the earth, they (men and women) managed to mess up again. They engaged in acts of evil, wickedness, and violence. Let's just say they were merely acting "human" and let their flesh take over. Unfortunately, as God watched from above, he was not happy with what he saw and responded by bringing a flood to destroy all flesh in which was "the breath of life" except for Noah, his immediate family and the animals confined in the ark Noah built (Genesis 6:17-19).

> *The Lord saw that the wickedness of man was great in the earth, and that every imagination and intention of all human thinking was only evil continually. And the Lord regretted that He had made man on the earth, and He was grieved at heart. So the Lord said, I will destroy, blot out, and wipe away mankind, whom I have created from the face of the ground — not only man, [but] the beasts and the creeping things and the birds of the air — for it grieves Me and makes Me regretful that I have made them.*
>
> *~ Genesis 6:5-7 (AMP)*

Yet, man's seed was eventually preserved thanks to the righteousness of one man: Noah. In God's eyes, Noah was just and righteous and walked in continual fellowship with God even though he was surrounded by a world of wickedness. Because of the favor Noah obtained from God, he received God's plan of action to preserve man's seed. Yes, God still destroyed every living thing on earth, but he used Noah to preserve the seed of all life forms. God had Noah save pairs of all animals and plant life, along with Noah's family.

Just as God commanded, Noah built an ark to protect them when the flood came. Afterward, God continued on with his original plan for man: "God blessed Noah and his sons, and said to them, 'Be fruitful and multiply, and fill the earth" (Genesis 9:1). This is interesting because it was the same commandment God gave to Adam and Eve long before the flood. You can assume that because this commandment is repeated, it holds a high level of importance to God.

Preservation and protection of the seed. That's what God is all about. He wants each and every family to multiply from generation to generation. This is yet another reason why children must be protected, especially in the area of eating. He also desires that you remain alive and healthy long enough to see your children's children (Psalm 128:6) and he wants you to have the pleasure of passing on a great lifestyle legacy to them.

Make no doubt about it. God loves our children too. He desires the best for them and expects parents to set a good course for their offspring so they may receive all the blessings he has in store for them. As a father figure, God set the course for the Israelites to depart from Egypt. He guided their travel from Egypt into Canaan using a cloud by day and a fire by night. After the Israelites had departed Egypt, they encountered many challenges along the way; it was not a perfect journey to say the least. However, God took care of them and led them from mark to mark and from glory to glory. His desire for us is expressed in Psalm 115:14, "May the Lord give you increase more and more, you and your children."

So, I (Kristy) encourage you to take inventory of your life today. In what direction are you leading your children? What kind of food are you feeding your family? What kind of food are you personally responsible for bringing into your household? Are those foods damaging your health, as well as the health of your family? Do you plan to be around to see and enjoy your children's children? How would your family manage if you suddenly died of a massive heart attack caused by things you can control such as your diet and lack of exercise? How many children would you leave your spouse to manage single-handedly on a single income without you? Ask yourself if your lack of discipline in the area of eating could be potentially damaging to your family. Now ask yourself what you are going to do to change things.

Chapter Summary

1. Children are the seed of each family. God desires the seed be protected, even when it comes to diet.
2. Children are falling prey to the damaging effects of processed foods.
3. It is parents' responsibility to ensure their children receive proper nourishment at home and away from home.

Chapter Fifteen

Filthy Lucre

No one can serve two masters; for either he will hate the one and love the other, or he will stand by and be devoted to the one and despise and be against the other. You cannot serve God and mammon (deceitful riches, money, possessions, or whatever is trusted in). ~ Matthew 6:24 (AMP)

At the outset of his ministry in Galilee, Jesus spoke the words above to teach his disciples a lesson on possessions and masters. He explained how it is impossible to operate effectively in God's kingdom if you idolize money and things. Kingdom-minded Christians should be faith-driven and not money worshippers. Seeking to attain and hoard wealth and material possessions any way you can, despite the impact on others, is a clear indication greed has taken over.

Could the food industry learn a thing or two from Jesus? I (Kristy) think so. On the surface it might seem as if the food industry giants are able to effectively serve both mammon and their customer base. Don't be fooled. They do not have your best interests in mind. If they did, sickness and disease would not be linked to the manufactured food and beverage products the industry makes available to you. Think about it. If you ran a company, would you sell a product you knew was responsible for making your customers sick, or worse?

In this day and age, you can no longer remain ignorant to the fact that the food industry is not operating with the primary intention of providing good, nutritious food to you and your family. You must stop assuming workers in food manufacturing plants or the butcher at the meatpacking facility are looking out for your nutritional needs. I hate to burst your bubble, but there are no "cooks" at these factories, wearing aprons and putting love into the food just like dear old mom. Instead, from my past experience in the food industry, interacting with product development teams, marketing teams, and a whole host of other people who knew little if anything about nutrition, I am aware of their true objectives. Their job is to concoct a product that will appeal to your senses, tickle your taste buds, take your hard-earned money, and make sure you came back to buy more. High demand, low production costs, and repeatedly high sales are always the objectives.

So, if providing you with nutritious food products and protecting your health is not top priority, what exactly is driving this lucrative industry? Money! As with any corporation, these companies' quarterly profit and loss statements are of paramount importance. Shareholders have a lot invested and are expecting substantial returns. For this reason, profit is the motivator. Your health is not the top priority. "For the love of money is the root of all kinds of evil, for which some have strayed from the faith in their greediness, and pierced themselves through with many sorrows" (1 Timothy 6:10).

As President Calvin Coolidge said, "The business of America is business." To understand the heart of the processed foods business, you have to comprehend how the U.S. economy works; the concept is not hard to grasp. Businesses employ both labor and capital to produce goods or products. These firms then bring their enormously diverse wares to market, where they try to sell them to about 300 million U.S. consumers — not to mention customers in other parts of the world.

While there are many company players who represent a multitude of industries, they all compete in the same game. Businesses want to sell their products for the highest price possible and consumers want to buy them as cheaply as the producer will permit. Each participating firm wants to gain some advantage over its competitors so they will capture consumer dollars. Whether the business is a manufacturer of toys, cars, lawn mowers, or cosmetics, the motives are the same. In order to be in business and to stay in business, your attention must be on making a monetary profit.

All stages of the food production process have proven to be fruitful, including the manufacturing, packaging, and distribution of food at the grocery store level. In fact, food companies fight for shelf space and aisle positioning in supermarkets. Often paying premiums, sales agents are driven to get their respective products on the shelves faster and to get them placed more prominently than the competition. Unlike the fruit and vegetable stands of yesteryear, food is now being distributed in unconventional ways. Buying in bulk is the economical way to go. People can purchase memberships to wholesale clubs whereby they can secure two-month supplies of cookies, crackers, soft drinks, and toilet paper all in one shopping trip. This lure of reduced prices has convinced many people to adopt a lifestyle of a squirrel wherein hoarding is strongly encouraged.

Given the large amounts of money consumers spend, you have to sit back and wonder what exactly are they buying. I (Kristy) took note of this on a routine trip to the supermarket. Because I had twelve items, I was polite and did not go into the "Ten Items or Less" checkout lane. Instead, I got in line behind people who had grocery carts full of stuff. I use the word "stuff" because, according to my training, the things I saw in the cart of the lady in front of me could not possibly be classified as "food."

As I waited patiently to pay, I was uncomfortable watching this woman purchase a cartload of items that quite possibly were going to put even more weight on her already well-endowed frame and potentially clog up her arteries, paving the way for a future heart attack or stroke. Frozen pizzas, frozen pies, pre-sweetened cereal, 2 percent milk, white bread, two gallons of ice cream, chips, frozen microwave meals, pork chops, frozen cookie dough, and two cases of diet soda were among her selections. I did not see any fresh fruit or any fresh vegetables in her cart. As much as my heart wanted to intervene and stop her from buying those things and doing further damage to herself and possibly her family, I knew my hands were tied. The nutritionist in me wanted to give her some unsolicited advice to help her but I knew it was not the time or the place.

It is not an accident that Americans are becoming obese and sickly because of an over-consumption of items that have been proven to be detrimental to our health. So the question must be asked at some point: If all of these food items are known to cause obesity and can lead to sickness and disease, why are they still being produced? Better yet: Why are we still buying them? The answers are right under our noses.

Let's begin with the first question. The answer is money. Again, it's a simple law of economics. Businesses make money when they have a consumer base to which they can sell goods. Food is necessary for survival. We all have to eat. Therefore, the market potential for the food industries is virtually unlimited, making it a very lucrative business. Expanding your market is a basic business strategy. That's why McDonald's began extending its market into China after receiving government approval in 2004. Adding as many as 120 restaurants a year was a key component of its plan to boost profits. Many other fast food and processed foods companies have followed suit.

But will the diseases so common in the West become more prevalent among people in the Far East as a result? According to a 2006 Associated Press article, approximately sixty million Chinese (equal to the population of France) are now obese. The article includes comments from Pan Beilei, a deputy director with the government-affiliated State Food and Nutrition Consultant Committee who reportedly said, "An increasing number of Chinese are eating more fat and junk food but less grains and vegetables, leading to a high number of cases of high blood pressure and diabetes." ("60 Million Chinese Are Considered Obese", Associated Press, November 6, 2006). Because of poor eating habits, according to Chinese Ministry of Health statistics, 160 million Chinese had high blood pressure in 2005, up from 90 million in 1991, and 20 million had diabetes.

To answer the second question, we have to study the demographics of the buyers. Whether they are Caucasian or Asian, young or old, short or tall, the majority of consumers have one thing in common: they are uneducated on the types of foods the body needs to maintain optimal health and they have no idea how much damage certain ingredients and food products can inflict upon the body when consumed over a period of time. As a result, this naïve bunch continues to purchase unhealthy foods blindly, day after day, month after month, and year after year. I am often surprised when someone confides in me that they were recently diagnosed with diabetes and that they can't figure out how they contracted the condition, as diabetes does not run in their family. With a sympathetic heart, I have to hold my breath to keep from saying, "Diabetes may not run in your family, but it probably does hide out in your kitchen pantry and refrigerator freezer."

While the majority of U.S. buyers are essentially clueless when it comes to shopping and eating healthfully, there is a small segment of consumers that is taking a more selective route when shopping for food. Some members of the 78 million baby boomer population are actively seeking ways to slow down their aging process. These methods include modification of diet and regular exercise. Apparently a light bulb came on in the heads of many boomers about 20 years ago. At that time an article entitled "Eat, Drink, and be Healed," reported that more than 80 percent of adults aged twenty and older said they were aware of health problems associated with eating behavior and being overweight. (*American Demographics,* March 1988). Unfortunately, we are not seeing enough fruit these days from this generation's efforts to be healthier.

This increased awareness of how nutrition affects health is why some Americans seem to be changing their diets, or at least considering the nutritional content of foods they buy. According to the *American Demographics* article, when people were asked if nutrition is an important factor in a food purchase, 70 percent of women and 54 percent of men said yes. In fact, 93 percent of adults eighteen and older say they are making some kind of change in their diets. The problem is the public is not very well versed on the best changes that should be made and can be fooled at times. In America alone, 49 percent of consumers want to learn more about the medical benefits of food.

So with this newly emerging group of consumers starting to break away from the traditional ways of the "Standard American Diet," what are processed food companies to do, knowing they will start to lose a percentage of their profits as people become more health conscious? The old motto "If you can't beat them, join them" applies here. A few of the industry's giants have taken a step outside the box by either purchasing health food companies or partnering with them. These profit-motivated moves are meant to protect their image as well as retain a segment of their market share that is making an attempt to slip away to the healthier side of life. For example, PepsiCo bottles water under the Aquafina brand while Coca-Cola has its Dasani water. Phillip Morris (Kraft Foods) purchased Boca Burger, a manufacturer of soy-based burgers. In addition, General Mills bought organic food companies Muir Glen and Cascadian Farms.

I (Kristy) was quite surprised one day when I used a dollar off coupon to purchase a new brand of soymilk I had not tried before. My incentive to buy was the coupon. The brand was 8th Continent and I found it to be much too sweet for my palate. One glance at the ingredient listing revealed there are two sugars in the product. Did the milk really need to be that sweet? After studying the additional coupon I received at the checkout line I found the manufacturer of the soymilk was none other than General Mills. Again, the traditional players are jumping in the game, but it seems they don't' understand all the nutritional rules.

A quick tour through some company web sites reveals how they are trying to make money off of the health-consciousness movement. These processed food companies are making an attempt to provide nutritional advice and teach families how to eat. Quaker has an on-line "Strive for Five," a five-step family nutrition program developed by Quaker in collaboration with the American Dietetic Association, which has ties to processed food companies. Kraft Foods takes it one step further. They have a section on their Web site totally dedicated to healthy living, featuring both a meal and fitness planner. They offer meals from Kraft's product line and a list of exercises meant to help you burn calories. Of course, their meal plans consist of the same pre-packaged and preservative-laden foods. And since when is a food company entitled to give expert fitness advice? The message here is no matter how much of a "goody two-shoes" image the processed food industry tries to portray, they are still making money at the expense of our health.

If money is your motivator, you will do almost anything. While a few food companies have made an attempt to service the health-conscious consumer, most processors will stick to the market that butters their bread, both literally and figuratively. If the majority of people are accepting, buying, and eating quick-serve meals, then, by golly, that's what companies will continue to sell. If you were the CEO of Dreyer's, the biggest U.S. packager of ice cream and home of Edy's ice cream, and were earning about $1.2 billion in sales annually, would you change your focus? You might if you had a concern for public health; you wouldn't if you were only in it for the money. "For where your treasure is, there your heart will be also" (Matthew 6:21). The works of the food industry and the message I (Kristy) desire to convey to you can be summarized in one key passage taken from Kelly Brownell's *Food Fight* book:

> Food companies confront the paradox of claiming public health as their priority while knowing that profits increase when people eat more. If the nation moves to a healthier diet, some segments of the industry will benefit and others will suffer. But for the industry as a whole, lower food consumption will lower earnings. Business acts in self-interest and industry leaders must protect their jobs, so significant changes in diet are frightening.

Chapter Summary

1. The processed food industry is money-motivated; nutrition and your health are not their primary focus.
2. Poor quality food is produced because consumers continue to purchase it.
3. Consumers continue to purchase poor quality food because they are uneducated on the types of food the body requires to maintain optimal health.

Chapter Sixteen

Magic Bullets

***...and by your magic spells and poisonous charm all nations
were led astray (seduced and deluded).
~ Revelation 18:23 (AMP)***

While government agencies and food industry groups are telling us what to eat, pharmaceutical companies and doctors are telling us what pills to take to cover up the pain and other symptoms of poor health caused by what we eat. We take little to no responsibility for this area of our lives. Instead, we abdicate control of our health to those who make a handsome profit off our illnesses and ignorance. Over and over we eat things that hurt us and then go looking for a quick, painless fix. And that's exactly what the drug industry wants us to do. With over two billion prescription drugs dispensed each year, pharmaceuticals have proven to be a vital part of life for many.

Have a headache, heartburn, or stomachache? The common response is to pop a pill. Anything that makes the pain go away fast becomes a best seller. We are in a hurry to feel better and look better. Our desire for quick fixes paved the way for Xenical, the so-called "fat pill" for teens. This handy little drug is supposed to limit the body's ability to digest fat. At $1,500 for a year's supply with a prescription, it should come complete with a new wardrobe! Any parents considering this drug for their teenagers should really question this expense and this approach to weight loss.

But thanks to the FDA, those strapped for cash can still get access to this handy-dandy little capsule. In February 2007, the agency approved a milder version of the drug for over-the-counter sale. It's called Orlistat and is reduced to half the dosage of prescription Xenical. The drug's maker — GlaxoSmithKline — says Orlistat is expected to cost one to two dollars a day. Some experts call Orlistat's side effects "awkward." They reportedly include abnormal bowel movements with oily defecation. Dr. Sidney Wolfe, the director of Public Citizen's Health Research Group, called the FDA's approval of Orlistat "reckless," citing studies that the prescription version Xenical has been associated with precancerous lesions of the colon. (*Chicago Tribune* - February 8, 2007).

Despite these kinds of reports, our passion for pill popping continues. Some people take manufactured medicine for every little ache or pain. Others would rather take drugs as the answer to their health conditions instead of adopting healthy diets. Too many people in this country simply cannot imagine life without the various pills crowding their medicine cabinet. And that's exactly the mentality the drug companies want. They've even come up with a pill for overweight dogs! On January 5, 2007, the FDA approved a canine weight-loss drug called Slentrol. Pfizer, who estimates 40 percent of American dogs are obese or overweight, manufactures it.

In recent years, drug makers have pulled out the big media guns to push their products. In 1997, the FDA began allowing pharmaceutical companies to market certain pain medications directly to consumers. The drug companies took advantage of the opportunity — especially on nightly television. A *USA Today* article described the advertising bombardment this way:

> If aliens landed on Earth and watched TV for an hour, they'd no doubt conclude that Americans are the most drug-dependent creatures in the universe. Advertisements for prescription drugs are fired out like baseballs in a batting cage. Trouble sleeping? Take Ambien! High cholesterol? Try Zocor! Heartburn? Ask about Nexium!

We have all seen the television ads where the list of a drug's side effects is longer than its benefits. Viewers are urged to talk to their doctors about the medication. Like your doctor is really going to say anything bad — especially since some of their perks come from drug company representatives. Would you take a drug that has a side effect of death? A product with this word of caution exists on the market now, but the warning might be missed because it is listed in fine print.

According to the *Journal of the American Medical Association* (*JAMA*), these multi-colored pharmaceuticals are killing thousands each year. In a study published in 1998, researchers found adverse reaction to prescription drugs may rank somewhere between the fourth and sixth leading cause of death in the United States. The April 27, 1998, edition of *Newsweek* carried this excerpt from the *JAMA* report: "It has been documented that antihistamines, in combination with the wrong antibiotic, can lead to abnormal heart rhythms; in rare instances the result can be fatal. ... Blood thinners alone, for example, can cause fatal internal hemorrhaging." Heart disease and cancer may hold the top two positions in terms of leading causes of death, but who would have ever thought prescription drugs — which are perceived by the masses as being beneficial and curative — could be ranked as a cause of death among the world's deadliest diseases? By the way, taking pharmaceuticals does not typically cure disease. They generally merely suppress your symptoms, while the underlying condition remains.

In order to be classified as a pharmaceutical, a product must have some level of toxicity. *Merriam Webster's Online Dictionary* defines "toxicity" as: "Containing or being poisonous material especially when capable of causing death or serious debilitation; extremely harsh, malicious, or harmful." An LD-50 rating is applied to every drug, indicating the dosage amount above which the drug would kill 50 percent of tested lab mice.

From a spiritual standpoint, none of this should come as much of a surprise. The word *drug* comes from the Greek word *pharmaco*. *Hastings Dictionary of the Bible* defines "pharmacy" (*pharmakon* in Greek) as "magic charm, poison, drug; ...to practice magic." Some Bible scholars say *pharmakon* was used in the original Greek translation of the Bible but was translated as *witchcraft* in Galatians 5:20 of the King James version of the Bible and translated as *sorcery* in the New Revised Standard version. In Christian circles, anything connected to witchcraft and sorcery is bad news from a spiritual and physical standpoint. The bible makes it clear that those who engage in such practices create a barrier to having God's best. (See Galatians 5:19-21 and Deuteronomy 18:10-11.)

Given the hazards posed by some drugs available today, it wouldn't be hard to connect them to an image of a witch standing over a big pot brewing up a potion to destroy her enemies. Some of these modern day concoctions could appropriately be described as "magic bullets" because their contents are a mystery to the average person and because they can cause great harm, just like a bullet from a gun. Taking them could end up like a game of Russian roulette gone badly. But day after day people religiously continue to pop such pills like M&M candies.

The concept of people taking pills for their pain started out nobly enough. When the pharmaceutical industry was birthed in the United States after the Civil War, prescription formulations were quite different from what we see today. In the beginning, these businesses offered homeopathic remedies derived from herbs and plant extracts. "By the 1880s, newly formed companies with names like Merck, Abbot, and Eli Lilly were producing prodigious quantities of standardized preparations including bloodroot, barberry, mayapple, and salicylic acid, an aspirin precursor," says Kenny Ausubel in *When Healing Becomes a Crime*.

As time progressed, so did the industry. By the 1920s the pharmaceutical giants had changed their protocols. The practice of creating healing solutions with chemicals replaced the use of herbs and botanicals. "Big Pharma" realized it could make more money by owning a unique chemical blend and then marketing it as the sole solution for a particular ailment. Botanicals were naturally found in nature and were not patentable. This limited opportunities for long-term profitability. Because an herbal or 100 percent plant-based treatment cannot receive a patent, pharmaceutical companies had no financial incentive to continue to market them. Thus, the patented pharmaceuticals business began — establishing the foundation for the most profitable industry in the world. And America, the richest nation on the planet, has the dubious distinction of being the most lucrative prescription drug market on the planet.

Patents allow the manufacturer to have exclusive rights to market a drug for a designated number of years. If a company has complete patent protection, it also is at liberty to set prices based upon its liking, and not necessarily based upon the true cost to manufacture the drug. It is estimated profits from pharmaceutical companies exceed 16 percent, which is triple that of the average Fortune 500 company.

Unfortunately, as the drug industry grew, pharmacologists' understandings of the complexity of the systems of the human body did not. They became more like chemists, and less like doctors, in their massive brewing of toxic chemical substances promoted as an excellent option for managing your health. This very same practice continues today.

> Drug discovery was an industrial process as much as steelmaking or automobile making. Drug companies did not primarily study disease; they formulated thousands of chemical compounds annually. Pharmacologists did not labor to understand how a compound and a disease interacted — they sought to test as many compounds as they could to see what worked. The more money they spent, the more compounds they screened, the greater the probability of discovering the next penicillin. The drug industry was producing more new drugs not because it better understood underlying biological reality but because it had learned to

manipulate small molecules chemically and to organize screening more efficiently.

~ Kenny Ausubel, When Healing Becomes a Crime.

So that explains why taking multiple drugs may provoke a negative reaction when combined, or why drugs can cause an adverse reaction in the body. They were quite possibly developed by chemists who perhaps did not know as much about the intricacies of God's wonderful human design as they should given their line of work. And with all the money that's being made, there is no incentive to enhance their education in this area.

For many people, all was well with their meds until September 2004. That's when Merck pulled its blockbuster arthritis painkiller, Vioxx, from the market after its own study found a higher rate of heart attacks and strokes in patients taking the drug than in those on a placebo. *Time* magazine's October 11, 2004, edition called the news a "bombshell that rocked financial markets." Vioxx debuted to rave reviews in 1999. It was considered a giant among the pharmaceutical industry's most popular drugs. In 2003, Vioxx reportedly racked up $2.5 billion in worldwide sales and accounted for 11 percent of Merck's revenue.

When the Vioxx story broke, other pharmaceutical companies began "assuring" consumers their products were safe. Some drug companies took out full-page ads in newspapers claiming, "Patient safety is our number one priority," and giving more details about their pills than is commonly published in the media. Newspaper editorials posed ominous questions, such as, "Does another Vioxx lurk among your prescriptions?"

Shortly after the Vioxx story broke, competitor drug maker Pfizer went on the offensive to protect the profitability of its arthritis drug, Celebrex. To assure the public about the drug's safety, Pfizer put a full-page ad in *USA Today,* saying:

> Celebrex has been making people with pain and arthritis feel better for years. And now we want to ease your mind too. Celebrex is in the same general medicine class as Vioxx, but it's not the same medicine. Important patient studies with Celebrex show strong cardiovascular safety.

To further reassure the public, the Celebrex ad also included the results of various studies indicating their drug did not pose the same potential health problems as Vioxx. But a few months later, Pfizer updated that press release with information about Celebrex that was less than positive. The company announced the drug might cause heart problems if taken frequently in high doses. Pfizer lost $24.3 billion in market share when this news hit.

So whom can you trust? The drug manufacturers? The regulators? The U.S. government knows the food and drug industry needs better regulatory systems. You may ask, "What about the FDA? Isn't it supposed to make sure all food and drugs are safe before they are approved for sale to consumers?" Yes. The agency does have those oversight responsibilities. But, unfortunately, this watchdog for consumers seems to need its own watchdog or at the least a bigger staff.

In 2004, the FDA came under fire when one of its own blew the whistle. After the Vioxx issue surfaced, FDA scientist David Graham told a Senate panel his twenty-year employer was incapable of protecting the public from dangerous drugs. He called the FDA "insensitive to drug safety." Graham began telling all after he conducted a study of both Vioxx and Celebrex. The results made him talk loudly and often. He, too, found people using Vioxx had a higher rate of heart attacks and sudden cardiac deaths than Celebrex users. But the real noise started when Graham accused the agency of trying to get him to soften his conclusions. He said the FDA was trying to block his First Amendment right to free speech. FDA officials say the agency promotes open internal debate about scientific issues. But Graham was quoted as saying, "When you live in a climate of fear, retaliation and intimidation, no decision that one makes is entirely voluntary." (*USA Today*, 2004)

The Vioxx and Celebrex situations have focused a lot of attention on the FDA. Critics say the agency is too closely linked with the pharmaceutical industry. High-priced lobbyists are accused of persuading the agency to do its bidding. Another problem is a large part of the FDA's funding comes from user fees paid by the very companies seeking the agency's permission to market new drugs. In February 2005, after a year of debate on the dangers of these arthritic drugs, advisors to the FDA concluded the benefits of Vioxx and Celebrex outweigh their risks. The group voted to allow Vioxx to return to the market, suggesting the drug carry a very strong warning label.

The question for consumers is this: Why would an agency designed to protect the public from harmful food and drugs turn a blind eye to a medicine on the market when studies show it significantly increases the risk of heart attacks in patients? Is the organization overworked or underfunded, or are its leaders unaware or, even worse, just indifferent? Whatever the reason, the lesson in all of this is clear: Do not rely on the government to keep unsafe foods and drugs off the market. Rely on yourself to keep unsafe foods and drugs out of your body.

If the pharmaceutical giants and members of the healthcare industry were as concerned about our health crisis as they say they are, they would do more to promote prevention. Educating the masses on nutritional interventions could potentially prevent disease. Logical? Yes. Profitable? No, at least not as profitable as treatment. That's no doubt why we don't hear much discussion about correcting the root causes of disease. Our society just continues a cycle destined for disaster. People get sick with lifestyle illnesses. They go to the doctor. The doctor often prescribes pills to help the patient cope with the symptoms. Depending on the sickness, the doctor might "recommend" a change of diet and an exercise program. The patient ignores the fitness advice and runs to the nearest drug store. The pharmaceutical companies make money and continue pushing a culture that promotes treatment over prevention.

Take a look at cancer. This condition has created one of the most profitable industries in the health field. In 1971, President Nixon declared a war on cancer and subsequently allotted the largest budget in history to go toward medical research on this disease of somewhat mysterious origins. According to Ausubel in *Healing Becomes a Crime*, "While a small, concentrated circle of corporations holds the patents on cancer drugs for private profit, most of the research funding to develop them has come from taxpayer dollars, through the federal government and the National Cancer Institute (NCI). The NCI has been dispensing a budget averaging $1.5 billion a year since the 'War on Cancer' began, with much of the largesse channeled to private corporations and research dollars."

Nixon's declaration was one in which he assured the nation cancer would be defeated. Take a look around. The battle is being waged with intensity today. While the United States continues to spend more than $1 billion per year on cancer, it seems improbable a cure has not been found to date. Actually, history has tucked away the truth.

A cure for cancer was discovered as far back as 1924 when Harry Hoxsey founded the first Hoxsey Clinic in southern Illinois. Using a combination of herbs including barberry, buckthorn, burdock root, cascara sagrada, licorice root, pokeroot, and red clover (straight from God's garden), Hoxsey devised a successful, non-toxic herbal formula pivotal in the treatment of over 25,000 people who had been afflicted with cancer. People would flock from all over the world just to receive the ray of hope Hoxsey had to offer. African-Americans, as well as the Christian community, heavily supported his work. Hoxsey based the cost of his treatment on what his patients could afford to pay, often administering his services for free. He eventually relocated his clinic to Texas, where it became the world's largest privately held cancer center with branches in seventeen states.

Would Hoxsey's treatment be worth billions today? Perhaps, but who knows? Posing a hypothetical question is all we can do, thanks to "Big Pharma," other traditional healthcare industry groups, and the government. For years, Hoxsey pleaded with organized medicine to review and test his formulary, hoping it would receive national recognition as a standard of care for cancer. "Condemnation without investigation" prevailed, and, unfortunately because Hoxsey did not have "M.D." after his name, coupled with other financial considerations, key players who should have been on his team — the American Medical Association (AMA) and the FDA— met his treatment with much resistance. These two powerful entities collaborated in driving Hoxsey and his treatment out of the United States by the mid-1960s, forcing him to go to Tijuana, Mexico, to continue his version of a plant-based treatment.

Knowing about the history of Hoxsey and how many disregarded his cancer solution, I (Kristy) am appalled by the intense marketing efforts that exist today, urging consumers to provide financial support "in search of a cure." Hogwash! Every spring I usually am solicited to financially support a 5K run for a cure or a three-day walk for breast cancer. The request no doubt comes from someone who has a very sincere heart and good intentions. My refusal to sign their pledge form stems from the failure to get an answer to this question, "Where does all the money go?"

Our financial support of ineffective organizations and our personal resistance to taking preventive measures to maintain good health has turned the mass treatment of cancer into a very lucrative industry. The big bucks are made from the *treatment* of the disease, not its prevention. (This holds true for some other diseases, too.) Think of all the business professionals involved in the management of a single cancer patient — the oncologist, the primary care physician, the chemotherapy technician, the pharmacist, the pharmaceutical manufacturer, the laborers in the pharmaceutical manufacturing plant, the scientists … the list goes on and on. It has been said if a cure for cancer were ever publicized and adopted by the masses, it would upset the economy and send this nation into a depression.

The reality is disease does not happen just by chance. Whether the condition is pink eye, stomach flu, or cancer, a cause exists. Therefore, the only way to find the solution or cure for cancer is to look at the cause. If the causes are removed, then the disease can be arrested. Unfortunately, our U.S. healthcare system is not designed to teach you the causes of disease and how you can avoid contracting many of them. Why should they? They only make money after you become a patient. If prevention were practiced, there would be no patients and the American healthcare system would look vastly different from a financial standpoint.

It is important to understand that "conventional prevention" is quite different from God's preventive methods. Some of the preventive measures suggested by mainstream medicine should be placed under scrutiny. In his book, Ausubel says, "Around 78,000 people a year get cancer from medical and dental X-rays. In just one generation, the number of cancers caused in this way is estimated around 2.3 million. ... One Canadian study found a 52 percent increase in breast cancer mortality in women given annual mammograms, a procedure whose stated purpose is to prevent cancer." These are not preventative procedures. They are nothing more than a "look see" to determine if a person has been unfortunate enough to get this horrible disease.

The same is true of recommendations encouraging women to have their breasts removed before breast cancer is even diagnosed. Why is this done? Because it fits the standard protocol for addressing cancer that's been around since the 1950s — stop it or prevent it with: surgery (cutting out the tumor), radiation (burning out the tumor), and chemotherapy (killing the tumor with chemicals). However, these methods are not as effective as they are promoted to be by the experts. It is estimated over a million people a year receive chemotherapy.

But according to Ausubel even an official with the National Cancer Institute (NCI) went on record some time ago identifying its downside:

> "Chemotherapy combinations can significantly raise the risk of secondary tumors" (Cancer Principles and Practice of Oncology). "Note: This is the standard textbook that was written by the former director of the NCI. ... Virtually all the chemotherapeutic anticancer agents now approved by the Food and Drug Administration for use or testing in human cancer patients are (1) highly or variously toxic at applied dosages; (2) markedly immunosuppressive, that is, destructive of the patients' native resistance to a variety of diseases, including cancer; and (3) carcinogenic. (Statement made by the head of the NCI Cytochemistry Division, Dr. Dean Burk, in 1973.)

Could prevention be an alternative to chemo? It would no doubt cost a lot less. If everyone would wake up and take a proactive approach, perhaps there would be one less funeral you'd have to attend this year. But "real" prevention starts with us.

In a *Success* magazine article entitled "Supernutrition vs. Cancer: The Best Offense is a Good Defense," Dimitrios Trichopoulos of the Harvard Center for Cancer Prevention said, "Cancers of the lung, breast, prostate, colon, and rectum become more frequent in countries where risk factors such as cigarette smoking, unhealthful dietary habits, and exposure to dangerous chemicals at work in the environment are now more common. Only diet rivals tobacco smoke as a cause of cancer in the U.S., accounting for a comparable number of fatalities each year. More than half of the cancer deaths in the country — perhaps even 60 percent — can be attributed to tobacco smoke and diet." (*Success*, January 1998). Even the National Academy of Science says most cancers are related to the "Standard American Diet," which consists largely of hot dogs, white bread, and coffee. Our cure can be found in what we avoid as opposed to what pill we take.

Thus, our lifestyle choices drive two major industries: food and pharmaceuticals. As God's children for whom he desires prosperity and health, we have the authority to reshape one of these businesses and reduce or eliminate the need for the other. But will we exercise that authority? Only time and statistics will tell. The money we spend fighting the results of our own ignorance and food excesses could be better spent to take the gospel of the kingdom throughout all the world as Jesus commanded. Let's redirect the wealth so the movement of money in the marketplace lines up better with God's plans for all our lives.

Chapter Summary

1. Dependency on pharmaceutical drugs has become a way of life for most Americans, Christians included.
2. Today, all pharmaceuticals have a level of toxicity creating a possibility for side effects and adverse reactions.
3. Pharmaceuticals do not cure; they merely treat "symptoms".
4. Our improper diet drives the pharmaceutical industry.
5. Preventive practices, including healthy eating, are the best way to keep unsafe drugs out of your body.

Chapter Seventeen

Kingdom Nutrition

Let your food be your medicine and your medicine be your food. ~ Hippocrates, 390 A.D.

It was as predictable as a rainstorm on a hot, humid day in July. Every Sunday, you could wager your most prized possession on the fact the battle would take place. The attack was not a large scale, hostile war fought between countries over issues such as political policy or the debated use of nuclear warfare. Nor was it a matter of a televised sporting event, where two boxers took turns throwing punches at each other with the intent of causing severe pain or unconsciousness. By far, these battles are much too complex in comparison to the weekly scrimmage in which I (Kristy) chose to partake.

The battleground? My parents' kitchen table. The weapons? They were simple instruments: knives and forks. I sat on one side of the table and my parents sat directly across enemy lines. My siblings remained on the sidelines, merely observing the repetitive face-off. One would think the bout had been televised the weekend before and what was being shown was an instant replay. My younger brother and older sister chose not to get involved in the contest and did not dare support either party. Perhaps they did not want to deal with the consequences of being perceived as a traitor defecting to the enemy camp. In their eyes, the event was a small clash with a quick resolution. In my eyes, it was a war of monumental significance. I put up my best fight. I stood my ground. I was not going to budge no matter what the enemy (my parents) instructed me to do.

Unfortunately, it was a tug of war I lost every Sunday, as this was the day my mother made a huge spread of soul food. The standard fare was macaroni and cheese, whipped sweet potatoes, pot roast with gravy, over-cooked greens, milk, white bread with butter, and strawberry shortcake for dessert. Mom would spend all afternoon in the kitchen, mixing, cutting, baking, and tasting the many delicacies she would present with love and honor to us each and every Sunday at five p.m. Because our weekdays were filled with sporting events and music recitals, we did not always have the pleasure of dining together as a family during the week. Mom put forth an honest effort to make up for this each Sunday. I assume it was her way of giving us a "treat" — a way of providing some form of compensation for the bologna and cheese sandwiches we often ate during the week.

This Sunday meal was also Mom's way of reinstating her position as the caretaker of the family. How she managed to work a full-time job as a nurse, often called away to the hospital during holidays, and raise six children (seven, if you count my dad!) is beyond my scope of comprehension. There is something to be said for the modern day version of the industrious wife and mother described in Proverbs 31. While I am positive my other family members looked forward to the feast with great anticipation, I dreaded the very thought of being called to the dinner table. In fact, I know my pace was slower than molasses as I descended the stairs on the way to the kitchen. Upon hitting the last stair and taking my assigned seat at the table, I knew the war was about to begin, and so did everyone else. Reflecting back on those times, I should have been shouting, "Let's get ready to rumble!" And my parents should have prayed for peace as they blessed the food set before us.

The Sunday meal would begin in silence. Bowls of food would pass from one hand to another, and each person would scoop several spoonfuls of starches and vegetables onto their plate. My plate showed more white space. A finicky eater, I would only grab what I knew I could stomach: bread and butter, macaroni and cheese, and a minute cut of pot roast. After selecting my buffet of three menu items, I would hear my mother's voice: "Kristy, get some greens." That was her call to action; I had to comply. Too bad Mom was not serving the only two vegetables I liked and was able to swallow with minor pain: peas and string beans.

As the meal progressed, I would slowly eat everything on my plate, leaving the greens for last. I had tried them before and it wasn't pretty as I gagged on the wilted vegetation. I adopted the rule that anything that smelled bad and looked bad would never touch my lips again, regardless of how good it was supposed to be for me. While everyone else had cleaned their plates and was enjoying the thrills of eating strawberry shortcake with whipped cream on top (which I didn't like either), I would sit arrested, staring at the dead plant in the middle of my plate. Before long, my dad would speak. "You are not getting up from this table until you clean everything on your plate," he'd say. "Children in Africa are starving and you are sitting here wasting food!" Battle cry number two had been declared and served as an indicator the war was heating up.

Hours would pass as the battle continued. I would stand my ground with a stern look on my face. No matter how intense things got, I would not give in and eat something I did not like. Unfortunately, there was no leaving the scene of the battle unless I did. Looking at the clock, hours would pass. A five p.m. dinner would turn into an eleven p.m. sit-in. Abandoned on the battlefield, I sat among the leftovers that had been neatly put away in color-coded Tupperware containers. No army buddies around for support. No secret rescue mission planned. Fearing the outcome, my siblings would yearn for me to give in and end the war just by taking one forkful of the greens. For me, it was an all-or-nothing situation; either I would give in and find a way to consume my vegetables, or just wait it out and deal with the consequences. The former solution was not an option to be exercised.

Suddenly, the war would come to an abrupt end. My parents' patience would subside, forcing me to throw in the white flag. My dad would re-enter the kitchen and announce a final command, thus ending the hostile situation. I would lose the battle, just as in the previous week, and would be instructed to march upstairs and receive my punishment — a spanking. Sometimes I got the belt, other times I was reprimanded with a homemade paddle. Nevertheless, it was painful. Afterward I would be sent to the barracks, jumping into my bottom bunk only to cry myself to sleep.

Sound painful? Looking back it was. All that drama just to avoid eating vegetables! Many would ask, "Was it worth it?" To me ... absolutely! At the time, I did not understand the value of nutrition. All I knew was the greens looked, smelled, and tasted horrible; therefore, I was not interested! I put Brussels sprouts, cabbage, cooked carrots, and lima beans in the same category. I wish I had known back then what I know now. I did not know the greens contained chlorophyll, which is a major cancer fighter in the body. Nor did I know the greens contained fiber, which is essential for cleansing the digestive tract. No wonder my parents were adamant that I finish off what was on my plate — although I doubt they really understood the specific nutritional reasons at that time.

The ability to understand the significance of making correct eating choices is crucial to combating Satan in this war on health. God has already given us a strategy to follow. It is simple, doable, foolproof and far superior to any plan devised by man in these modern times. The world's system has all types of food pyramids and calorie-counting protocols, which unfortunately do nothing but lure people into making incorrect food choices that do not support an overall condition of good health. Everywhere you go, someone has a different opinion on what constitutes healthy food and what does not. One day the media tells you drinking coffee daily is healthy for you and the next day the same news outlets report spinach is dangerous because of an E. coli outbreak. The question is this: Whose dietary standard will you follow? God's or man's? Wisdom dictates that you follow the manufacturer's maintenance guidelines. Ignoring God's directions on how to keep your body healthy is like buying a Lexus and taking advice on maintaining this luxury vehicle from a bicycle repairman instead of a mechanic for Toyota, the Lexus manufacturer.

Nevertheless, television commercials, billboards, and self-appointed health gurus out to make a fast buck tell us how to eat. And we go willingly to the trough, letting our taste buds guide our choices. As a result, hamburger joints and coffeehouses all across America do a brisk business. People hold these places in great esteem and worship at them daily. Have you ever noticed how you never have to drive far to find one? These handy little franchises are strategically located in every neighborhood.

The fast food industry influences U.S. dietary habits to the tune of more than $110 billion a year, which is what consumers spend on fast food. This is more than the amount spent on personal computers, computer software, new cars, and higher education combined, according to Eric Schlosser in *Fast Food Nation*. The fact that Americans go on diets eighty million times a year should tell you there is something about our current eating lifestyle that is just not right.

How do we fix it? By going to the best source available for guidance on what foods we should be eating. That source is the same Creator who designed our bodies. He knows exactly what nutrients we need to stay healthy and made sure the meal plan was memorialized in writing. This operating manual is for everyone — man, woman, boy, girl, Christian, and non-Christian. It's called the Bible.

I (Kristy) often refer to the bible as our Basic Instructions Before Leaving Earth. Within God's written Word, he has provided all the policies and procedures we need to overcome life's trials and tribulations while we are here on planet earth. It contains instructions on personal conduct, good business practices, financial prosperity, how to pick a mate, how to raise children, and even how to eat. God knew if we were left to our own devices, we would mess up the simple matter of eating right. So, he gave us some instructions for healthy eating. Many of them are found in the Old Testament. Some of you reading this book right now may already be saying to yourself, "But we are not under the Old Testament Law anymore; we are under a New Covenant." Yes, I (Kristy) understand your rationale. However, your thinking is incorrect. Just as we should not ignore the truths of the Ten Commandments, we should not ignore God's Old Testament dietary or health laws.

Thank God for the New Covenant. It is through the death and resurrection of Jesus Christ that we are able to receive healing and wholeness from our poor eating habits, but if we give strict adherence to the original laws, we can avoid many health calamities. Since it was God who created man, it should be obvious that he would know how best to take care of his creation. So, regardless of *where* the instructions for healthy eating are provided in the Bible, they are important instructions from the Maker himself and should not be disregarded.

Starting in the book of Genesis, God provides the first instructions on how to eat. For God to make mention of this in the first chapter, he must have felt it was a topic of high priority. The initial verses of Genesis record how God spent six days creating his masterpiece of a universe. After creating a firmament called heaven, it was on the third day God created earth and then decided to adorn it. "And God said, 'Let the earth bring forth grass, the herb yielding seed, and the fruit tree yielding fruit after his kind, whose seed is in itself, upon the earth': and it was so. And the earth brought forth grass, and herb yielding seed after his kind, and the tree yielding fruit, whose seed was in itself, after his kind: and God saw that it was good" (Genesis 1:11-12 KJV).

Like an interior designer selecting wallpaper and paint to decorate a home's interior, God was selective in his choices for adorning the earth with food products. His decision to cover this world with plants, seeds, and fruit was precise and carefully carried out. These three items are referenced in Genesis 1:11-12. Included in the category of herb yielding seed are whole grains and beans. The last sentence of this Scripture summarizes God's point of view on his creation: "God saw that it was good."

If the foods created were not categorized as being good, then God would not have made them available to people. Man did not come on the scene until Genesis 1:27. After Adam's creation, he is then presented with the gifts from God's garden and is told to consume them for meat. Understand that in this context, the word *meat* means food or nourishment — it has nothing to do with animal flesh. God informs Adam in Genesis 1:29-30 that he has already prepared and provided the nutrients that will be needed for health and longevity.

So what does the Bible say about healthy eating? While there are many Scriptures on this subject, I (Kristy) will focus on eight primary food categories referenced in the Bible and intended for nourishment (notice processed foods did not make the list!): fruit, vegetables, meat, beans, whole grains/bread, nuts/seeds, good fats (olives/olive oil), and honey (dessert).

Fruit and Vegetables

And God said, Behold, I have given you every herb bearing seed, which is upon the face of all the earth, and every tree, in the which is the fruit of a tree yielding seed; to you it shall be for meat. And to every beast of the earth, and to every fowl of the air, and to every thing that creepeth upon the earth, wherein there is life, I have given every green herb for meat: and it was so. ~ *Genesis 1:29-30 (KJV)*

In these two foundational Scriptures, God outlines what the staple should be for our diets today: fruit and vegetables. It is imperative to consume these foods in abundance if you are to attain and maintain health. God provided in fruit and vegetables the key nutrients needed to sustain life.

And every plant of the field before it was in the earth, and every herb of the field before it grew: for the Lord God had not caused it to rain upon the earth, and there was not a man to till the ground. But there went up a mist from the earth, and watered the whole face of the ground.
~ *Genesis 2:5-6 (KJV)*

Before the first rain fell upon the earth, God caused a mist to cover the face of the earth and water the seeds and the herbs while they were yet in the ground. I honestly believe it was in this mist that essential vitamins, minerals, and enzymes were deposited in the soil in which vegetation was to grow. Once again, God knew what he was doing. Hence, he prepared the soil to provide the plants with the nutrients man was going to need; he made provision before man was even formed. And even prior to making the provision, he made the commandment for us to eat of the foods he was preparing.

Did you have a piece of fruit or a salad today? Don't answer. But you should not let a day go by without eating fruit and vegetables, as they are the "spice of life." The specific nutrients within fruit and vegetables were designed by God to cleanse our body and to provide healing. "At least two hundred epidemiological studies from around the world have a link between a plant-rich diet and a lower risk for many types of cancer," says Stephanie Beling, M.D., in *Power Foods*. Sadly, most people consume fruit a few times a week and hardly any vegetables. If they do eat a vegetable, most often it is iceberg lettuce, which has little to no nutritional value. When correcting my diet, I (Kristy) used the guidelines provided by Dr. Don Colbert in his book *Toxic Relief* in order to increase my intake of fruit and vegetables. At a minimum, I try to consume two fruits and three vegetables a day. Colbert calls this "Five Alive."

Every fruit and vegetable contains specific phytonutrients; some refer to them as phytochemicals. Derived from the root "phyto," which means "plant," phytonutrients are substances that occur naturally in plants and they have the ability to prevent and combat disease. Phytonutrients are essentially a plant's very own antioxidants produced to protect the plant from the internal damage or oxidation that occurs while it is converting sunlight and carbon dioxide to form oxygen so we can all breathe. This process is referred to as photosynthesis. Not only do the phytonutrients in plants protect the plant, they protect us as well if we consume such vegetation. Note the healing power of these categories of phytonutrients.

- *Chlorophyll:* leafy green vegetables, wheat grass, blue-green algae, barley grass, spirulina. Contain anti-viral, anti-tumor, and anti-oxidant properties. Chlorophyll is found only in green plants and combats tumor growth.

- *Carotenoids:* apricots, carrots, tomatoes, strawberries, mangos, oranges, peaches, nectarines, red grapes. Are antioxidants that help the cells differentiate between cancerous and non-cancerous cells. Carotenoids have been shown to decrease the risk of heart disease as well as various types of cancer. They boost the immune system and offset macular degeneration.

- *Flavonoids:* eggplant, cherries, blueberries, blackberries, grapes, plums, peppers, white pigment inside the peel of citrus fruits. Help to prevent heart disease and blood clotting. Help to prevent your skin from breaking down (sagging and wrinkling).

- *Isothiocyanates:* cauliflower, broccoli, Brussels sprouts, cabbage, kale, greens. The most powerful cancer-fighters available. Stimulate the production of enzymes that break down carcinogens (cancer-causing agents) in the body.

- *Organosulfur Compounds:* onions, garlic. Inhibit tumor growth, help to cleanse the blood, decrease blood-clotting, and lower cholesterol. Garlic and onion may block the formation of nitrosamines, which are cancerous compounds that can form in the digestive tract.

Interesting, huh? The world's system is spinning its wheels and spending countless dollars looking for a cure for cancer while our heavenly Father has provided a preventative plan through fruit and vegetables. Instead of living in fear of this dreadful disease, you can take a less-expensive, more offensive approach to warding off cancer by selecting food components from God's "farmacy."

Notice fruit and vegetables are kept in the "produce" section of the grocery. Perhaps it is because these foods are designed to "produce" life. Broccoli, cabbage, red peppers, yellow squash, orange potatoes, blueberries, raspberries, yams, and red beets offer God's life-yielding nutrients. And the colors of these items are symbolic as well. The presence of phytonutrients in fruit and vegetables is marked by the bright, colorful hues found in the skin — the same colors found in the rainbow. Why?

In Genesis, God used the rainbow to mark a covenant with Noah.

> *And God said, This is the token of the covenant (solemn pledge) which I am making between Me and you and every living creature that is with you, for all future generations: I set My bow [rainbow] in the cloud, and it shall be a token or sign of a covenant or solemn pledge between Me and the earth. And it shall be that when I bring clouds over the earth and the bow [rainbow] is seen in the clouds, I will [earnestly] remember My covenant or solemn pledge which is between Me and you and every living creature of all flesh; and the waters will no more become a flood to destroy and make all flesh corrupt. ~ Genesis 9:12-15 (AMP)*

The rainbow was God's visual reminder that he would never use floods to destroy the earth. This was not only a covenant made between God and Noah, it was a contract between God and future generations as well. The New King James version uses the term "perpetual generations" to explain the longevity of the agreement. Hence, the rainbow is a reminder that God desires to bring life and not death and destruction. Think about this when you are shopping for groceries. The products in the produce section are designed to bring life and I (Kristy) believe for that reason they have been assigned a unique color from the rainbow.

To receive the true benefits of fruit and vegetables, consume them in their raw state. This means not cooking the vegetables until they are mushy and not eating canned fruit swimming in sugary syrup. Additionally, many people would argue that consuming bottled fruit juices is the same as eating raw fruit. This is another myth to dispel. Similar to the process of over-heating vegetables, fruit is over-heated when it is bottled. This occurs during the pasteurization process, which is performed to kill off bacteria in bottled juices. Not only do the bacteria die, the active enzymes you require for nourishment are mutilated as well. Bottled juices contain too much concentrated sugar, usually as high fructose corn syrup, a highly processed and fattening sugar added to the fruit juice.

Feeling heavy and bloated? Fruit is important because it is the cleanser of the body. Fruit is loaded with two components necessary to ensure our colons work consistently and efficiently: fiber and water. Fiber is found within the fruit's skin. Fiber, or roughage, is the broom that sweeps waste out of the digestive tract and out of the body. Studies have shown that incidences of colon cancer and other digestive disorders are very low in populations with high-fiber diets. Industrialized nations where diets are high in fat and low in fiber have high incidences of these diseases. Water is within the core of fruit. Water is essential to sustain life and for proper colon function.

Meat

While Adam and Eve were provided an abundance of fruit and vegetables to eat in the Garden of Eden, it was after the flood that God made an amendment to his original dietary law and allowed for animal meat to be eaten for the first time. God also instilled an instinct in animals causing them to fear man.

> *And God blessed Noah and his sons, and said unto them, Be fruitful, and multiply, and replenish the earth. And the fear of you and the dread of you shall be upon every beast of the earth, and upon every fowl of the air, upon all that moveth upon the earth, and upon all the fishes of the sea; into your hand they are delivered. Every moving thing that liveth shall be meat for you, even as the green herb have I given you all things. But flesh with the life thereof, which is the blood thereof, shall ye not eat. ~ Genesis 9:1-4 (KJV)*

The newly established law allowing man to consume meat as a source of food for the first time was now public policy and the animals knew it as well. Today, we are permitted to consume meat but it is to go "along with" our vegetables. Genesis 9:3 suggests, "Every moving thing that liveth shall be meat for you, even as the green herb have I given you all things." Thus, green herbs (vegetables) should go on our plates first, and meat should be the side dish, not the other way around. We often pile meat on our plates and use a small portion of vegetables as the side dish.

It is important to clarify that a completely vegetarian diet, where no animal protein is consumed at all, is a recipe for poor health. The body requires protein, carbohydrates and good fats daily, and animal protein is the richest source. The bible warns us about those who tout the extreme eating plans of today such as vegetarianism and veganism:

Now the Spirit speaketh expressly, that in the latter times some shall depart from the faith, giving heed to seducing spirits, and doctrines of devils.

Forbidding to marry, and commanding to abstain from meats, which God hath created to be received with thanksgiving of them which believe and know the truth. ~ I Timothy 4:1,3 (KJV)

While a vegetarian diet is not a requirement for optimal health, our consumption of poor quality meat from fast food establishments and chain restaurants should be minimized. Americans continue to uphold the customary standard of having meat (particularly red meat) with at least one meal every day, contributing to obesity and colon problems because meat contains no fiber and may take anywhere from three to four days to exit the body. Biblical diets did not allow for this. Red meat was consumed primarily on special occasions. When the prodigal son returned home in the Luke 15, his father wanted to celebrate. Not only did he clothe his long-lost son with his best festive robe of honor, he also proclaimed, "Bring hither the fatted calf, and kill it; and let us eat, and be merry" (Luke 15:23 KJV). Similar to a modern day birthday cake, the red meat delicacy was permitted because a joyous event was taking place.

Of all the meats available, fish was the one on which very little restriction was placed. The Gospel of Luke gives an account where Simon received an abundance of fish after following radical instructions from Jesus to go fishing during the daylight hours.

Now when he had left speaking, he said unto Simon, Launch out into the deep, and let down your nets for a draught. And Simon answering said unto him, Master, we have toiled all the night, and have taken nothing:

nevertheless at thy word I will let down the net. And when
they had this done, they inclosed a great multitude of fishes:
and their net brake. ~ Luke 5:4-6 (KJV)

In John 6, Jesus performed yet another miracle in order to feed his followers. Using two small fishes and five barley loaves from a young boy, Jesus multiplied the meal and was able to feed five thousand people with fish and bread. No doubt the Hebrews realized the dietary benefits of having fish at mealtime. Eating three to four ounces of fish on two or three days a week instead of red meat will assist in reducing the risk of heart attacks and strokes because fish — specifically cold-water varieties such as halibut, mackerel, salmon, and sardines — provide essential omega-3 fatty acids that help to thin the blood, lower cholesterol, and lower blood pressure. Omega 3 fats are also critical for proper brain function, which affects vision, learning ability and retention, muscle coordination, and mood. Depression and anxiety are two mood disorders that can result from a lack of omega 3s.

Two additional guidelines about meat consumption were established in the book of Leviticus. We are instructed not to consume the fat portion of meat or raw meat that still contains blood.

It shall be a perpetual statue for your generations throughout
all your dwellings, that ye eat neither fat nor blood.
~ Leviticus 3:17 (KJV)

Speak unto the children of Israel, saying, Ye shall eat no
manner of fat, of ox, or of sheep, or of goat. And the fat of
the beast that dieth of itself, and the fat of that which is torn
with beasts, may be used in any other use: but ye shall in no
wise eat of it. For whosoever eateth the fat of the beast, of
which men offer an offering made by fire unto the Lord,
even the soul that eateth it shall be cut off from his people.
Moreover ye shall eat no manner of blood, whether it be of
fowl or of beast, in any of your dwellings.
~ Leviticus 7:23-26 (KJV)

Leviticus 3:17 uses the word *perpetual* again, meaning "continuing forever." God initiated a statute forbidding fat for all generations. The fat referenced in Scripture is saturated fat, or fat that comes from animals and not plants. While this type of fat was not to be eaten, it was acceptable for sacrificial purposes. It was often the fat surrounding the kidneys and intestines that was burned by the priests.

God knew what he was doing. He makes no mistakes. He says in Leviticus 7:24 that you are wise if you do not consume the fat of any meat. Because cattle are now raised on fattening grains instead of grass, their fat content is far greater than the meat of biblical days — something that must be considered when planning your meals. Routine trips to the local hamburger joint could put you in line for heart disease down the road. Seek to purchase grass-fed/grass-finished beef which is extremely lean. This type of beef is not detrimental to your health because the cattle have been fed grass throughout their entire life-cycle.

He also provides wisdom for avoiding raw meat or meat that has been half-cooked, whereby blood is still flowing. The blood is the lifeline of any species. This is noted by Rex Russell, M.D., in his book, *What The Bible Says About Healthy Eating*, who says, "Scientists have long known that blood carries infections and toxins that circulate in an animal's body. If people eat animal blood (raw meat), they are needlessly exposed to these infections and toxins."

In addition to establishing guidelines around the parts of meat to be eaten, God also clarified the types of meat we are to eat. In Genesis 7:2, God classifies animals into clean and unclean groups: "Of every clean beast thou shalt take to thee by sevens, the male and his female: and of beasts that are not clean by two, the male and his female" (KJV).

He gave a purpose to each classification. Unfortunately, the unclean animals have been given the responsibility of cleaning up the waste and toxic matter here on the earth. These scavengers are considered dirty and are not suitable for food.

> *Whatsoever parteth the hoof, and is clovenfooted, and cheweth the cud, among the beasts, that shall ye eat. Nevertheless these shall ye not eat of them that chew the cud, or of them that divide the hoof: as the camel, because he cheweth the cud, but divideth not the hoof; he is unclean to you. ~ Leviticus 11:3-4 (KJV)*

These shall ye eat of all that are in the waters: whatsoever hath fins and scales in the waters, in the seas, and in the rivers, them shall ye eat. And all that have not fins and scales in the seas, and in the rivers, of all that move in the waters, and of any living thing which is in the waters, they shall be an abomination to you. ~ Leviticus 11:9-10 (KJV)

Say goodbye to Red Lobster. No more pork chops – not even once a week as a Sunday treat. It is important to accept that the following items are not on the list of meats and seafood acceptable for human consumption: pork (bacon, sausage, pork chops, chitterlings), catfish, lobster, shrimp, oysters, clams, squid, escargot, crabs, and scallops. Because of their eating patterns and lack of sweat glands by which toxins are normally released, pigs consume parasites, bacteria, viruses, and toxins that are then passed on to humans. Shellfish can be referred to as "filters of the sea" or "bottom-dwellers." These sea creatures span the bottom of the ocean, filtering large volumes of water daily. Sewage laden with chemicals, toxins, bacteria, parasites, and viruses become concentrated in these shellfish. As we eat the flesh of the shellfish, we consume these very same harmful contaminants and disease-causing organisms.

While God's dietary guidelines may appear to be strict and nit-picky to some, there is a reason he took great measure to lay down these laws. He had our health in mind. "For I am the Lord your God: ye shall therefore sanctify yourselves, and ye shall be holy; for I am holy: neither shall ye defile yourselves with any manner of creeping thing that creepeth upon the earth. For I am the Lord that bringeth you up out of the land of Egypt, to be your God: ye shall therefore be holy, for I am holy" (Leviticus 11:44-45 KJV). God desired that we not defile our bodies so that through our actions we could remain a holy, separated people. Our bodies are to be a living sacrifice to God at all times. We all know that in making a sacrifice, it is necessary to forfeit or give up something. Sorry folks but that lobster tail has got to go!

Beans

Brought beds, and basins, and earthen vessels, and wheat, and barley, and flour, and parched corn, and beans, and lentiles, and parched pulse. ~ 2 Samuel 17:28 (KJV)

Then Jacob gave Esau bread and pottage of lentiles; and he did eat and drink, and rose up, and went his way: thus Esau despised his birthright. ~ *Genesis 25:34 (KJV)*

Beans were a staple item during biblical times and there is a good reason why. Beans are loaded with fiber, iron, and calcium. Their phytonutrient mixture marks them as tremendous cancer fighters and antioxidants, in addition to being effective in thinning the blood and reducing cholesterol. God gave us several different varieties of beans from which we are free to choose. Red beans, kidney beans, lentil beans, black beans, garbanzo beans, and navy beans … take your pick and simmer them in broth for soup.

A popular spread that is a common part of the Mediterranean diet is hummus. Hummus is made from crushed chickpeas, olive oil, and various seasonings; it is usually eaten with vegetables, crackers, or pita bread. When shopping for hummus, be sure to avoid brands that are made with processed oils such as canola and vegetable/soybean oil. The high-temperature processing of these oils causes them to "become rancid or oxidized, forming free radicals. These chaotic, skewed fatty acid molecules wreak havoc on the body, attacking and damaging DNA/RNA, cell membranes, vascular walls, and red blood cells; all of which may lead to deeper physiological damage, such as tumor formation, accelerated aging, arterial plaque accumulation, autoimmune imbalances, and more." www.wellbeingjournal.com, *Fats: Safer Choices for Your Frying Pan & Your Health,* July/August 2010.

Whole Grains/Bread

And Melchizedek king of Salem brought forth bread and wine: and he was the priest of the most high God.
~ *Genesis 14:18 (KJV)*

And he pressed upon them greatly; and they turned in unto him, and entered into his house; and he made them a feast, and did bake unleavened bread, and they did eat.
~ *Genesis 19:3 (KJV)*

And Boaz said unto her, At mealtime come thou hither, and eat of the bread, and dip thy morsel in the vinegar. And she sat beside the reapers: and he reached her parched corn, and she did eat, and was sufficed, and left. ~ *Ruth 2:14 (KJV)*

And Jesse said unto David his son, Take now for thy brethren an ephah of this parched corn, and these ten loaves, and run to the camp to thy brethren. ~ 1 Samuel 17:17 (KJV)

Many types of whole grains were eaten in biblical days. In fact, bread was a daily staple. Grains such as millet, spelt, barley, and rye provided essential vitamins and minerals, protein, and fiber to an active Hebrew culture. Today, wheat is the most common grain consumed with approximately 30,000 varieties grown throughout the world.

Yet, wheat is not the only grain from which we are to nourish our bodies. In fact, most available wheat products are heavily processed and are essentially white flour products providing little nourishment. Some lesser known whole grains include quinoa, amaranth, and buckwheat, which can be used as a side dish instead of potatoes and rice, and are far better for the body. All of these grains provide necessary fiber, which helps to maintain proper colon function and cholesterol levels, and also provides a long-term fuel supply so you don't go hungry. The book of Ezekiel provides the formula for a power-packed, whole-grain bread called Ezekiel Bread: "Take thou also unto thee wheat, and barley, and beans, and lentils, and millet, and fitches (spelt), and put them in one vessel, and make thee bread thereof, according to the number of the days that thou shalt lie upon thy side, three hundred and ninety days shalt thou eat thereof" (Ezekiel 4:9 KJV).

The story behind the birth of Ezekiel bread is that a trained priest from Jerusalem named Ezekiel ended up in Babylonian captivity in 597 B.C. While he was imprisoned, God spoke to him and told him to be the "watchman" for the house of Israel. He was assigned the prophetic responsibility of taking the Word of God given to him and sharing its warning messages with Israel. One such message he was to deliver was regarding the siege of Jerusalem. This unfavorable report was to be presented by Ezekiel in the form of a skit. As part of the act, Ezekiel was instructed to lie down on his left side for 390 days to depict the iniquity or sins Israel had committed. He also was to lie down on his right side for forty days to play out the sins of Judah.

Symbolically, Ezekiel bore the punishment Israel was to eventually suffer. To sustain him during this trying period, God provided Ezekiel with the recipe for a mixture of grains and beans, which was to be eaten by weight — twenty shekels (a half-pound) a day. This meager meal represented the food rationing that would take place during the military siege. While the bread portion was small, Ezekiel was able to maintain his health and walk after spending more than one full year lying down! There is something to be said for beans and grains. A modern version of this bread is available today in most health food stores.

You will often find whole grain breads tucked away in the freezer section of the grocery store. Be on alert — if you find a loaf of enriched bread packaged nicely and neatly and left to sit on a store shelf for weeks and weeks, then it is essentially "dead bread" and should remain exactly where it is.

The whole grain category also includes pasta and rice. Avoid white pasta and white rice, as they have the same nutritional deficiencies as white bread. Instead, seek brown rice varieties for both rice and pasta dishes.

Nuts/Seeds

And their father Israel said unto them, If it must be so now, do this; take of the best fruits in the land in your vessels, and carry down the man a present, a little balm, and a little honey, spices, and myrrh, nuts and almonds.
~ Genesis 43:11 (KJV)

And it came to pass, that on the morrow Moses went into the tabernacle of witness; and, behold, the rod of Aaron for the house of Levi was budded, and brought forth buds, and bloomed blossoms, and yielded almonds.
~ Numbers 17:8 (KJV)

I went down into the garden of nuts to see the fruits of the valley, and to see whether the vine flourished, and the pomegranates budded. ~ Song of Solomon 6:11 (KJV)

Tree nuts come in many varieties, such as pecans, almonds, walnuts, and cashews. Nuts are another source of protein and, because they are a source of essential fatty acids (good fats) they are beneficial in improving heart health. Nuts and seeds provide linoleic acid (omega-6 fatty acid), which is beneficial in lowering cholesterol levels. Just snacking on a small handful of nuts in between meals can help to stabilize blood sugar levels, making nuts a much healthier snack food than cookies, potato chips, and pretzels. Seeds such as sunflower seeds, sesame seeds, and pumpkin seeds make a healthy complement to salads.

To get the most benefit from nuts, they should be consumed in their raw state. This means no salt, no sugar, no honey roasting, and no yogurt or chocolate coating. Almost every type of nut is beneficial except for peanuts and pistachios. Peanuts actually are not even classified as nuts but as legumes, and are difficult to digest. Additionally, both peanuts and pistachios tend to contain a great deal of mold.

Good Fats (Olives/Olive Oil)

Command the children of Israel, that they bring unto thee pure oil olive beaten for the light, to cause the lamps to burn continually. ~ Leviticus 24:2 (KJV)

A land of wheat, and barley, and vines, and fig trees, and pomegranates; a land of oil olive, and honey.
~ Deuteronomy 8:8 (KJV)

Thou shalt have olive trees throughout all thy coasts, but thou shalt not anoint thyself with the oil; for thine olive shall cast his fruit. ~ Deuteronomy 28:40 (KJV)

Olive oil is used extensively throughout the Bible. Not only was it used to light candles and for anointing, olive oil also was consumed quite often with meals. Our ancestors recognized the body requires the good omega-9 fatty acid found in olive oil. Like the other sources of good fats found in nuts and fish, olive oil is one of the best. In *What The Bible Says About Healthy Eating*, Rex Russell, M.D, says, "The Greek people, who consumed large amounts of olive oil, had an extremely low incidence of hardening of the arteries. Further research has shown olive oil is digested like complex carbohydrates and has healthful fatty acids, which is actually a windfall for health — particularly for a vascular disease such as hardening of the arteries." An easy way to take in olive oil is to make it a part of your salad dressing. A mixture of balsamic vinegar, seasonings, and olive oil makes for a tasty dressing. Most health food stores now carry salad dressings with an olive oil, rather than vegetable oil, base.

Honey

My son, eat thou honey, because it is good; and the
honeycomb, which is sweet to thy taste.
~ Proverbs 24:13 (KJV)

And they gave him a piece of a broiled fish, and of an
honeycomb. ~ Luke 24:42 (KJV)

He should have fed them also with the finest of the wheat:
and with honey out of the rock should I have satisfied thee.
~ Psalm 81:16 (KJV)

Stay me with flagons, comfort me with apples: for I am sick
of love. ~ Song of Solomon 2:5 (KJV)

God did give us a palate for something sweet, but it was not for refined cane, beet, or corn-based sugars, nor for the synthetic, chemically manufactured sweeteners such as Equal, Sweet'N Low, and Splenda we find in our grocery stores today. Rapidly digested refined sugars may in fact provide a quick form of energy, but their frequent consumption has contributed to the rise in conditions such as hypoglycemia, diabetes, and obesity, all resulting from the body's inability to maintain proper blood sugar balance. "All forms of concentrated sugar — white sugar, brown sugar, malt, glucose, refined honey, and syrup — are fast releasing, causing a rapid increase in blood sugar levels. If this sugar is not required by the body it is put into storage, eventually emerging as fat. Most concentrated forms of sugar are also devoid of vitamins and minerals, unlike the natural sources of fruit," says Patrick Holford in *The Optimum Nutrition Bible*.

Instead, we were designed to favor the natural sweetness of fruit (fructose) or unrefined, raw honey. Both fructose and raw honey are classified as slow-releasing sugars (low glycemic), meaning they do no provoke a rapid increase in blood sugar levels. Raw honey, specifically the darker honey, contains beneficial vitamins and minerals, as well as calcium, magnesium, phosphorus, and potassium. It also has various enzymes and amino acids that aid in digestion.

So the next time you find yourself developing a sweet tooth and want to treat yourself to a homemade dessert, consider using raw honey instead of refined sugar in your recipe.

While a treat from time to time is permissible, the Bible also provides a warning about overindulging on sweets (even the natural ones), so please take heed.

Hast thou found honey? Eat so much as is sufficient for thee, lest thou be filled therewith, and vomit it.
~ Proverbs 25:16 (KJV)

It is not good to eat much honey. ~ Proverbs 25:27 (KJV)

Isn't it awesome that God loved us so much that he designed an eating plan for us to follow? His eating plan consisted primarily of foods derived from the earth or suspended from a vine or a tree. God did not provide food manufactured in a factory. Only such items as automobiles and washing machines are manufactured. Food is grown — or at least in theory it should be. So the next time you are shopping in a grocery store, walk down the aisle with a new set of eyes. Ask yourself if ingredients such as artificial flavorings, chemical colors, and synthetic sugars are God's best. If your answer is no, leave the product on the shelf and head straight to the produce section.

Chapter Summary

1. Because of his love for us, God provided dietary guidelines in the Bible.
2. God identified acceptable foods for us to consume: fruit, vegetables, meat, beans, whole grains/breads, nuts/seeds, good fats (olives/olive oil), and honey.
3. Each of these foods provides a source of nourishment to help maintain the human body as God intended.

Chapter Eighteen

Pay Now or Pay Later

My rich dad often said, "There are only two things you can invest: time and money." He also said, "Since most people do not invest much time, they lose their money."
~ Robert Kiyosaki, Why We Want You to Be Rich

It was 1995 and I (Kristy) had just moved from Minneapolis to Chicago. Leaving the cold, frigid temperatures of Minnesota for an environment that was on average ten degrees warmer during the winter season was worth the move, in my opinion. When I arrived in the Windy City, I opted to live in a suburb just west of downtown. That first week I spent most of my time trying to bring some semblance of order to my condo. I then realized it was time for me to stop living off fast food and make the dreaded trip to the grocery store. The fridge was sanitized and ready to be stocked. Although I was new to the area, I vaguely remembered a grocery store I had passed a few days before called Whole Foods, so I made my way over to this market that was foreign to me.

Initially, I thought Whole Foods was just another little neighborhood store; unbeknownst to me, it was a national health food chain on the brink of rapid growth in its stock price. I wandered through the aisles feeling as if I was walking through the jungles of *Jurassic Park*. I saw oversized carrots and beets, and the colors of all the vegetables were much brighter than normal. Even the lettuce was different. Instead of finding nicely rounded heads of light green iceberg lettuce, I saw bins of various breeds of lettuces blended together — some green and some burgundy. It looked different, and I was too afraid to try it.

Leaving the produce section, I ventured over to the dairy aisle. I was able to find my 2 percent milk and my dozen eggs; however, the usual white eggs were next to cartons of brown eggs. I assumed the brown eggs must be bad, so I purchased a carton of the white Grade A eggs instead. Aisle by aisle, I managed to purchase most of the items on my shopping list, yet they were not my familiar brands. The bread was darker and heavier and was stored in a refrigerator instead of on the shelf. I was not able to find my favorite brand of cookies in the snack aisle and my pre-sweetened cereal was missing. I have to admit I was slightly disappointed not to be able to locate any cream-filled snack cakes or my customary choice of ice cream.

After selecting enough items to cover me for a week or two, I made my way to the checkout line. I had "guesstimated" my bill would not exceed $50, since I had only picked up a few things. However, when I heard the cashier announce, "Your total is $135.98," I almost got tears in my eyes. As I wrote out my check, I kept pondering what additional items I must have mistakenly dropped in my cart to force my bill to exceed $50. I couldn't figure it out. I grumbled under my breath, "This store should have been named 'Whole Paycheck' rather than 'Whole Foods,' " because paying that bill made me feel as if they were after my entire paycheck. With no questions asked, I humbly pushed my grocery cart to my car and put my two little bags of food in the trunk, followed by a somber drive back to my condo. "I will never step foot in that store again!" I said defiantly.

Since my initial visit to this organic health food store, I cannot count the number of times I have been back. I started showing my face again in 1997, which is the year I began to turn my life around by eating healthier. In fact, as part of my profession, I now take people who are becoming more health conscious on tours of the store so they will not be as confused and intimidated as I was on my first visit.

So, why is there so much hoopla about shopping organically? Some of you reading this may be thinking, "I've gone to those kinds of grocery stores before and they are too expensive! I'm a single parent with three kids to feed. I need the best bang for my buck, food that tastes good to the kids so they will eat it and not waste it, and something quick and easy to prepare since I work all day. I honestly don't feel the need to change where I shop. At my regular grocery store, I can get three frozen pizzas for five dollars. How can the prices at some organic grocery beat the family pack chicken meal I can get for $12.49 around the corner, or the wide variety of items available on the ninety-nine-cent menu at a my favorite hamburger joint?" Do not be deceived. The price comparisons are not as scary as they seem. Besides, your health is worth any additional cost you might end up paying.

There is a *huge* difference between organic food and the conventional food found at the local grocery. This distinction is of particular importance when it comes to fruit and vegetables. When a product is labeled organic, this claim guarantees it has been grown, handled, and processed according to strict production standards that reduce and eliminate the use of toxic pesticides and fertilizers, and that prohibit the use of genetic engineering (cloning of food), irradiation (applying radiation to the food), sewage sludge (fertilizer from animal or human waste), growth hormones, and antibiotics. The Tufts University *Health & Nutrition Letter* reported in February 2001: "The farmland on which organic crops are grown is prohibited from being treated with synthetic pesticides and herbicides for at least three years prior to harvest. Furthermore, farm animals raised under organic standards cannot receive antibiotics or growth hormones."

Fruit, vegetables, and meat grown or raised by conventional methods do not receive the same care or oversight. Are you aware of the overall legalized adulteration occurring with non-processed food such as fruit and vegetables? Adulterate means "to corrupt, debase or make impure by the addition of a foreign or inferior substance; to prepare for sale by replacing more valuable with less valuable or inert ingredients." (*Webster's New Collegiate Dictionary*, 1981). How does this happen to food?

Let's start with fruit. Similar to a sponge, fruit and vegetables are porous and can soak in the various pesticides and insecticides applied by farmers. Federal government reports have revealed more than one million children a day are exposed to unsafe levels of organophosphates, which are a group of insecticides that have the ability to harm developing brain and nervous systems in children.

Commercially grown peaches, apples, and grapes were found to put the greatest number of infants and children at risk due to unsafe pesticide residue levels. The Environmental Working Group, a not-for-profit research organization, also compiled a list of conventional fruit and vegetables highest in pesticide residues. That list includes apples, cherries, strawberries, celery, spinach, green beans, cucumbers, and bell peppers.

What about meat? If there is one food that should be purchased from an organic food store, it is beef and chicken. What is packaged and on display in a conventional store may look good to the eyes but the story behind those sirloin steaks and extra-large chicken breasts might curb your appetite. The mere manner in which the animals have been raised and maintained prior to packaging is the issue and the potential effect on human health is a serious matter about which the typical conventional grocery store shopper may not be aware.

In his book, *Diet for a New America,* John Robbins (of the Baskin-Robbins ice cream dynasty) documents how this multi-million dollar industry has changed over the years. He says:

> Increasingly in the last few decades, the animals raised for meat, dairy products, and eggs in the United States have been subjected to ever more deplorable conditions. Merely to keep the poor creatures alive under these circumstances, even more chemicals have had to be used, and increasingly, hormones,

pesticides, antibiotics, and countless other chemicals and drugs end up in foods derived from animals. The more unnaturally today's livestock are raised, the more chemical residues end up in our food. But that's just the half of it. The suffering these animals undergo has become so extreme that to partake of food from these creatures is to partake unknowingly of the abject misery that has been their lives. Millions upon millions of Americans are merrily eating away, unaware of the pain and disease they are taking into their bodies with every bite. We are ingesting nightmares for breakfast, lunch, and dinner.

What Robbins describes are the cattle and chicken factories where multitudes of livestock are kept in severely overcrowded conditions until slaughter. Let's take a quick look at conventional chicken production. These fowls are not raised in open chicken yards but are raised in cages. The average warehouse chicken flock is about 80,000 birds, and for an animal with strong territorial needs, these living arrangements are devastating. They are crowded into tiny cells, just as employees crowd into an elevator at five p.m. when it is time to go home. This is why the term "cage-free" on organic egg cartons is to be valued.

Inside the factories, the chickens are deprived of what they enjoy the most, which is natural light. The result is a group of birds that have no sense of a natural sleep cycle, and are literally driven crazy by the crowded and dark conditions. The environment is one of chaos where chickens fight for space and a natural desire to establish a social or pecking order. To prevent their early death and loss of profits, the chickens' beaks are removed.

It gets worse. What are the chickens fed during their imprisonment? Get this: Virtually all chickens raised in the United States are fed a diet of antibiotics from the time they are hatched. Hormones, antibiotics, nitrofurans, and arsenic compounds are all standard fare. (And you thought you weren't on any drugs?) Without antibiotics, the chickens could not be raised in massive quantities and company profits would be severely impacted. With these multitudes of hormones that are added, it is not coincidental that children today are experiencing abnormal growths in height and girth and women's hormonal issues are on the rise.

Despite the chemical efforts, the animals are full of disease. Chickens raised for their flesh, and not for their eggs, are sold by weight. So for these chickens, a healthy diet is really not a concern to the processors. Their job is to just fatten them up for the slaughter in the fastest and most economical manner possible.

> A government report found that over 90 percent of the chickens from most flocks in the country are infected with chicken cancer (leucosis). In fact, due to the danger of contracting diseases from chickens, the Bureau of Labor has listed the poultry processing industry as one of the most hazardous of all occupations. ~ John Robbins, Diet for a New America

If that's not enough, let's look at the beef production industry. It also uses non-traditional practices in raising cattle. They are fed grain as opposed to grass, and are loaded up with growth hormones to control disease in the crowded conditions in which they also live. The net result is hamburger and steak products in our supermarkets contain too much saturated fat and a bountiful seasoning of growth hormones and pesticides. Again, the human hormonal system does not stand a chance when this type of meat is consumed. A malfunction in this system of the body is inevitable.

You can minimize your worries about whether or not you are feeding your family hormone- and pesticide-laden chicken or beef by buying these items solely from a health food store. Will it cost more? Probably. Will it be better for you to eat chicken or beef without pesticides? Yes. Your body does not need these chemicals. Instead, buy grass-fed beef, organic chicken, and free-range eggs. (By the way, the eggs *will* be brown in color!) The meat policy at one health food grocery store I (Kristy) frequent makes the following guarantee regarding their cuts. The grocery has nothing to hide, as these guarantees are posted in the store for all shoppers to see:

- Fed a one-hundred-percent vegetarian diet with no animal by-products
- No added hormones or antibiotics
- Tractability of each animal back to their place of birth
- All cattle processed before twenty-four months of age
- No sick, lame, or "downer" animals processed into meat
- Freshly ground beef from whole muscle meat
- Mandatory third-party audits for food safety and humane animal treatment at the processing plants

Since conventional meat is not safe, you may ask, "What about other food items? Is there anything else for which I should be on the lookout?" Absolutely. Watch out for foods that contain genetically modified organisms (GMOs). Other commonly used phrases for these products are genetically engineered (GE), genetically modified, biotech foods, gene-foods, gene-altered foods, or transgenic foods. What are they? Genetically modified food has a genetic makeup that has been altered by combining DNA molecules from different sources. For instance, let's say you plant a garden with peas in it. Later you notice little bugs, called weevils, are eating your peas. You then hire a scientist to come up with something to make the weevils go away. Mr. Scientist goes into his lab and starts researching the problem. He learns beans have a protein molecule that will make it hard for the weevils to digest the peas. So the scientist combines the bean molecule with the pea molecule to grow peas that the weevil won't eat. The new and improved pea is actually a whole new "organism."

It all sounds very helpful and progressive, doesn't it? But what happens when Mr. Scientist starts combining plant life with animal life — such as a tobacco leaf with a gene from a firefly? Or the gene from a worm into chicken and cows so they can make their own omega-3 oils, which are heart-healthy substances commonly found in fish? Suddenly, that Porterhouse steak you love to eat doesn't sound so mouth-watering. The bottom line is some weird things can happen to our food long before it makes it from the field and the slaughterhouse to our tables. Much of it has been touched by the wonders of science and chemistry. This sounds like something from a science-fiction movie, doesn't it? Well get ready to enter the *Twilight Zone* of grocery shopping.

Walk through the aisles of any supermarket in America. Sit down to eat in just about any restaurant, school cafeteria, workplace lunchroom, hospital, or airplane. Open your cupboards and refrigerator. Look at what's cooking in your own oven, microwave, or frying pan, or what's on your fork, your spoon, in your cup or drinking glass. ... You can't see, smell, taste, or feel the difference. And you can't read about it on food labels or restaurant menus. But you and your family are now part of a vast culinary and biological experiment — dining on an expanding menu of genetically engineered foods. Foods that are unlike any foods consumed in human history. ~ Ronnie Cummins and Ben

Lilliston, Genetically Engineered Food: A Self-Defense Guide for Consumers

The authors of this book describe genetic food engineering as "the practice of altering or disrupting the genetic blueprints of living organisms, and humans — then patenting these altered genes and selling the resulting gene-foods, seeds, or other products for profit." It is nothing more than mankind's misguided effort to re-create food. But even worse, it is a scary attempt to play God with our food supply system.

Research on genetic engineering technology began in the 1970s. Twenty-five years later, scientists began experimenting with it to increase milk production in cows. They started injecting them with the recombinant bovine growth hormone (rBGH). In February 1994, at a cost of $500 million, Monsanto gained approval to take this genetic monster to market. The intent was to increase total milk production by 25 percent. But a definite downside to this hormone has been reported. "The single most disturbing aspect of rBGH from a human safety standpoint concerns Insulin-like Growth Factor-I (IGF-I), which is linked to breast cancer. IGF-I occurs naturally in human beings as well as cows, but rBGH injections cause substantial and sustained increases in IGF-I levels in milk sap," says Samuel S. Epstein, M.D., professor of occupational and environmental medicine at the Illinois School of Public Health, in Robert Cohen's *Milk: The Deadly Poison.* "IGF-I is not destroyed by pasteurization, survives the digestive process, is absorbed into the blood, and produces potent growth-promoting affects."

The net result of this test-tube creation is that cancer rates skyrocketed due to an increase in the production of the IGF-I hormone. After analyzing data from twenty-seven countries in the 1970s, Harvard Medical School was able to correlate milk consumption to increased rates of ovarian cancer. It is also believed to pose serious hazards for prostate and colon cancer. Yet, despite such reports, some of our most highly respected organizations — the American Medical Association, the American Diabetes Association, and the National Institutes of Health — continue to promote milk as necessary for good health. No one should be drinking milk for all the reasons cited in Chapter 14 of this book. But if you must have cow's milk, at least buy organic.

From milk, genetic food engineering has now exploded across a multitude of agricultural food items. Today, crops such as soybeans, corn, wheat, tobacco, cotton, tomatoes, rice, and potatoes have been genetically modified. Chances are it's in most of what you eat. According to the *Pew Initiative on Food and Biotechnology Fact Sheet,* "The Grocery Manufacturers of America estimates between 70 percent and 75 percent of all processed foods available in U.S. grocery stores may contain ingredients from genetically engineered plants. Breads, cereal, frozen pizzas, hot dogs, and soda are just a few of them." Other foods that may contain GMO components are corn chips, corn sweeteners, popcorn, margarine, cooking oils, salad dressing, baby foods, and infant formula. Field-testing is already underway for vegetables such as bell peppers, cauliflower, lettuce, onion, broccoli, and cabbage, and it is just a matter of time before these altered foods hit the produce section.

So how do you know if the cereal and vegetable oil in your house is from genetically modified crops or if the carton of milk, package of cheese, pint of yogurt, or the half-gallon of ice cream sitting in your freezer is derived from milk containing the rBST growth hormone? You don't know. And who knows if you ever will.

The FDA does not require safety testing for genetically engineered foods. And it announced in 1992 that special labeling for GE food also was not required. The September 2000 issue of *Food Technology* reported that only "if a new or modified food is significantly different from its conventional counterpart in composition, nutritional value, or safety, the difference in food would be a material fact. For example, if a new processing technique resulted in a significant decrease in the nutrient content or change in flavor, color, or other valued characteristic of a food, a label or statement would be required to inform consumers of that material fact."

It is no surprise then that most Americans remain clueless about all of this. "A poll of one thousand U.S. citizens published on December 6, (2006) reveals only a quarter realize they're eating GM food, and 60 percent have no idea it's in their diet," reported at www.newscientist.com. All you can do is arm yourself with the latest information, the determination to live a healthy life, and faith in God's ability to protect you.

Why are large biotechnology companies such as Monsanto and Novartis participating in the production of this laboratory food? It's obviously very profitable. But in a public relations effort, they say GMO technology is being used to create crops that grow faster and resist weeds and insects. They say this increases crop production, which can help address the problem of world hunger. Apparently the FDA, the U.S. Department of Agriculture and the EPA agree because genetic food engineering has been allowed to expand with few restraints.

What was initially a concept has now grown into a huge industry with a few key players running the show. In fact, there is actually a battle being waged over farmlands between the farmers and the producers of the GMO seeds. Traditionally, farmers purchase seeds for their crops and are entitled to save seeds for possible planting the next year. The rules of the game have changed with GMO seeds and the purchasing power of farmers is different now.

> A decision by the Supreme Court in 1980 overturned a 200-year prohibition on patenting living organisms, and human cell lines. Researchers and investors realized they could now "own" entire varieties of plants and animals, as long as they "discovered" them (i.e., mapped out their chemical gene sequences) and/or "invented" them (i.e., performed certain genetic or chemical alterations, no matter how slight, on the natural version of these living organisms). These life patents in turn give the patent holder a legally binding copyright over a seed or animal, enabling them to charge a "technology fee" to farmers who grow these plants or raise these animals, or a "licensing fee" to scientists who want to research these organisms. ~ Ronnie Cummins & Ben Lilliston, Genetically Engineered Food: A Self-Defense Guide for Consumers

Corporations now hold intellectual property rights to the seeds and plant varieties. In order for farmers to plant, they must "lease" the seeds from the seed company. A contract is signed between the two parties and the farmer is restricted from saving seeds for future planting. He must use all the seeds in one season and allow the seed manufacturer access to his fields at any time. The reality? Farmers have no choice but to go back to the supplier and purchase more expensive seeds every year. This economic cycle does not favor the small farmers who customarily saved and replanted seeds due to financial constraints.

Meanwhile, the question of the long-term effect on human health is one that has yet to be answered. Concerned scientists predict increases in food allergies may occur as more genes from a wide variety of plant species are mixed. In addition, the use of antibiotics that have been spliced into animal feed are speculated to cause an increase in human resistance to certain bacterial strains. This could explode into a serious problem on a very large scale. It's no wonder that insurance companies will not currently insure genetically engineered crops.

Then there's the potential environmental impact. According to Cummins and Lilliston in *Genetically Engineered Food*, "Researchers documented in the December 2, 1999, issue of *Nature* that toxins from genetically engineered crops are leaking into the soil through the plants' roots systems, damaging or killing beneficial soil micro-organisms, disrupting the soil food web." When plant soil becomes affected, so does the nutritional value of products grown. The stakes are high when choosing to grow genetically modified food. Unfortunately, it has become a mainstream industry and the United States is its global cheerleader. God could not possibly be pleased with this frightening manipulation of his original design.

But the rest of the world, including many so-called "starving" nations, have either cried out in protest against food cloning or passed laws to carefully control its availability. They say the world's hunger problem is no reason to clone food because there is nothing wrong with traditional agricultural production techniques. The real problem, they say, lies with food distribution as a result of political unrest. Countries other than the United States are questioning if GMO products contain harmful allergens, toxins, poisons, antibiotic-resistant genes, infective viral agents, and greater pesticide residues.

This type of food processing is under such scrutiny that most of the European countries, Canada, and Japan have placed partial to complete moratoriums on the import of U.S. GMO food products. They have chosen to do so because there is not enough information about the long-term affects. When they published *Genetically Engineered Food* in 2004, Cummins and Lilliston noted the following state of affairs at the turn of the 21st century:

> **European Union:** In January 2000, "the EU agreed to label all processed foods that contain at least 1 percent of genetically engineered soybean or corn. This policy applies to all fifteen EU member nations."

> **Greece:** In April 1999 they "banned the import of genetically engineered rapeseed or canola."

> **United Kingdom:** "The U.K. is also the only country that requires labeling of genetically engineered food in restaurants. All of Britain's major supermarkets have   banned genetically engineered ingredients from their brand name products."

> **Norway:** This "is the only country in Europe to implement a blanket ban on all genetically engineered foods and crops."

Spain: In May 1999, "Spain's largest supermarket chain, Pryca, announced a ban on all genetically engineered foods."

Australia/New Zealand: "In December 1998, the Australia-New Zealand Food Standards Council called for mandatory labeling of GE food."

Despite these bans and restrictions, biotech mega-companies continue to dominate the food industry. Since 1996, the U.S. has consistently planted more GM crops than any other country. According to the National Agricultural Statistics Services/USDA, in 2003, 81 percent of the total soybean crop was genetically engineered, 40 percent of the total corn crop, and 73 percent of total cotton crop. In 2003, 25 percent of the world's 672 million acres of land under cultivation consisted of GM crops.

Many of the producers of the food sold in healthy shops are aware of the GMO scare and have taken additional steps to separate their products from the others. They voluntarily label their food products to proclaim they are GMO-free. Look for this label when you shop for food at a conventional store. You won't see this label nearly as often as you see "high fructose corn syrup" and "partially hydrogenated oil." In fact, your search for the GMO-free label will probably be like looking for a needle a haystack.

Given all the statistics on the link between diet and disease, why would anyone want to keep buying unhealthy food? Because for most of America, nutrition is not the driver. Good taste is a key factor influencing our buying habits, along with cost and convenience. "When people create their internal balance sheet, unhealthy foods have high value and low cost, but healthy foods have high cost and lower value, making conditions ripe for overeating," says Kelly D. Brownell in *Food Fight*.

While the cost of organic food may seem to be a lot higher at the checkout counter, in reality, it does not cost more than conventional food. I (Kristy) know that sounds contradictory, but let me explain. In order to fully understand my blanket statement, you have to see the full economic picture. The price of organic food — as with any product — takes into account all costs associated with bringing it to the store shelves, particularly the labor costs. In an effort to ensure the future of this food and its seed supply, organic farming encourages crop diversity by using the rotational system of planting.

This is how farming is supposed to be done and it's not a new process. It's outlined in the Bible: "Six years you shall sow your field, and six years you shall prune your vineyard and gather its fruit; but in the seventh year there shall be a Sabbath of solemn rest for the land, a Sabbath to the Lord. You shall neither sow your field nor prune your vineyard" (Leviticus 25:3-4). Organic farming also promotes composting, which is the recycling of plant and animal waste into natural fertilizer, as opposed to synthetic, chemical fertilizers. The result is our water and air supplies are protected from further pesticide contamination. Because organic farmers do not use synthetic herbicides to control weeds, the weed control costs are higher and must be passed down. Overall, those who grow organic products must adhere to stricter production and organic certification standards that govern systems such as growing, harvesting, transportation, and storage. All of these processes are time and labor intensive and, therefore, more expensive.

The cost of organic food actually could be reduced substantially if all of the perks of conventional food production were passed on to organic farmers. I'm talking about farm subsidies. The only reason conventional food is cheaper is because the U.S. government pays farmers subsidies for the raw ingredients. If you are not aware of how the government is subsidizing our major farm crops, now is the time to become informed because the effect on the price of your processed grocery store items is quite significant.

An agricultural subsidy is a government subsidy paid to farmers to assist them in supplementing their incomes. Subsidies can be granted in many forms, such as tax reductions, direct cash payments, and below-market prices on water or other inputs necessary to produce crops. Franklin D. Roosevelt first sanctioned the subsidies during the Great Depression to bail out struggling farmers who were in dire straits. Subsidizing was a good idea back then, but today subsidizing is deemed unnecessary and counterproductive by many hardworking taxpayers.

Here's how it works. By law, the U.S. Agricultural Department is required to subsidize over two dozen commodities, including corn, cotton, soybeans, wheat, tobacco, dairy, rice, and peanuts to name a few. It is estimated Congress shells out our tax dollars to the tune of $20 billion to $30 billion annually, with over 65 percent distributed to large corporate farms not in real need of the funding. The large farms and agribusinesses receive large donations, while the small, struggling farms receive little. Many of the handouts go to Fortune 500 companies including John Hancock, Northwestern Mutual Life, MeadWestvaco, Chevron, Caterpillar, International Paper, Eli Lily, Kimberly-Clark, and Navistar.

The reality of subsidizing is it guarantees a set minimum price for a crop, and the subsidized price is often higher than the true market value of that particular crop. For instance, a bushel of wheat could be valued at three dollars, yet the government could ensure payment of $3.50 per bushel through subsidies. This being the case, farmers often are encouraged to over-produce in an effort to get the additional kickback on their commodities. From an economics standpoint, when the availability of product exceeds market demand, prices drop and remain low. And that is exactly what the government wants. Sounds ludicrous, doesn't it? The government gives farmers our taxpayer dollars so we can buy back their raw ingredients in the form of processed cereals, sugar, cakes, pies, and snack items, yet at a reduced price. The farmers benefit because they receive more from the government than what they would in the free market. Sounds like a form of corporate welfare!

The problem is farmers of only select commodities are eligible for subsidy distribution. You see, it is the type of crop, and not farmers' income levels or poverty standards, which determines how farm subsidies are delegated. According to the website www.heritage.org, "Growers of corn, wheat, cotton, soybeans, and rice receive more than 90 percent of all farm subsidies; growers of nearly all of the other four hundred domestic crops are completely shut out of farm subsidy programs. Further skewing these awards, the amounts of subsidies increase as a farmer plants more crops."

Growers of traditional things like corn and wheat are subsidized, while farmers of fruit and vegetables are not. Is that fair? Absolutely not. Libby Quaid best summarized the reality of this inequity in a 2005 Associated Press article, "Feds Aren't Subsidizing Recommended Foods":

> Subsidies encourage an abundant supply of corn, wheat, rice, and soybeans. Much of the corn and soybeans is fed to livestock. Some is also turned into nutrition-poor ingredients in processed food for people. For example, toaster pastries contain partially hydrogenated soybean oil that gives them a flaky texture, and they contain high-fructose corn syrup to sweeten their fruit filling. That translates to lots of calories, lots of artery-clogging fat, and little or no fiber.

The same article quoted Adam Drenowski, professor of epidemiology at the University of Washington, who said, "If we tell a family, 'You really ought to be eating more salads and fresh fruit,' and this is a low-income family, we're essentially encouraging them to spend more money."

On a larger scale, subsidizing can be deemed wasteful. Remember when your parents told you to eat everything on your plate? Well, the government feels differently and actually encourages food wasting. Excess crops are produced and anything that doesn't make it to market is dumped or left in storage to rot. "According to The Institute for Agriculture and Trade Policy ... dumping rates are approximately 40 percent for wheat, between 25 and 30 percent for corn (maize), approximately 30 percent for soybeans, 57 percent for cotton, and approximately 20 percent for rice," according to *Agricultural Policy*.

The long-term environmental and health costs associated with pesticide and chemical fertilizers on conventional food items, as well as the global economic effect of farm subsidies, are not to be overlooked. While conventional food may appear to be cheaper and more affordable for us now, we will pay the price down the road. If we don't live to pay the price, our children will. They either will be plagued with obesity or stricken with a disease resulting from a lifestyle of consuming toxin-laced food and being exposed to them through our water supply system. Bottom line: you pay for what you get, although sometimes — just like with a credit card — your payment is deferred.

Ask yourself, "Do I value my body enough to spend more money to give it the best food available or would I rather save a few dollars now and then pay thousands more later when I am dealing with sickness and disease?" The University of California Berkeley's wellness newsletter reported a study found families saved money by switching to natural unprocessed food. After a year, they were spending much less than they did before the study began — and were healthier! In fact, 90 percent of most food people buy is processed, which is usually 200-500 percent more expensive than unprocessed foods.

Deciding to pay money for healthier food is like learning to tithe. Think about it. Do you remember when you were a new believer and first heard about the biblical principle of giving 10 percent of your paycheck to the "storehouse"? For most people, this is a hard teaching to accept. Depending on how large or small your check, a 10 percent deficit right off the top could put a serious damper on your monthly budget. Some of you may have kicked and screamed when the collection plate was passed but eventually gave it a try, just as God suggests in Malachi 3:10-12.

This teaching came to mind one day when I (Christine) was in a health food store. I wanted some organic spinach. When I saw the price, I actually said aloud, "I'm not paying $3.99 for some spinach!" Immediately, a still, quiet voice in my head said, "You pay your tithe, don't you? You bring it to the storehouse." I thought, *Well, yeah, but that's different.* But the still, quiet voice continued: "Then why won't you tithe into your physical storehouse?" Enough said! I bought the spinach and went home.

Just as there are benefits from tithing (blessings poured out from open heavens, preservation of your possessions, safety from the devourer), there are benefits from spending money on organic food. You are blessed with better health. Your temple is preserved for God's purpose. And you show the world a better way to live. Think of it this way: each time you spend money on conventional food, you are investing in an industry that still has a lot of questions to answer about the food it cooks up in a test tube and rushes to market. Eating organically is an investment in *you* — God's chosen vessel! So the next time you are shopping for food or eating out, stay on the alert. It is not just a mundane chore, but also a campaign against the forces that would rather keep you in the dark about the stuff being passed off as "food."

Don't throw up your hands in frustration wondering, "What in the world am I supposed to eat then?" Take this information and use it to better control your diet. Don't give up and say, "Whatever!" That's exactly what Satan wants you to do! Use your faith to consider the complex issues surrounding our tainted food supply. Seek God's wisdom. Decide now to overcome any fear you may have about what is happening to our food supply, worries that "health food" won't taste good, and concerns about the cost of these foods. Remember, "God shall supply all your need according to His riches in glory by Christ Jesus" (Philippians 4:19).

Chapter Summary

1. There is a significant difference between conventional and organic food.
2. Organic produce and meat are free from pesticides, herbicides, fungicides, hormones, steroids, and genetically modified components, all of which are harmful to the body.
3. We should be willing to spend more to give our bodies the best food available.
4. Forgoing the purchase of higher quality food now may result in paying a higher price later.

Chapter Nineteen

Severed Supplies

George Washington, the history books tell us, was beset by many enemies during the winter of 1777-1778 — including the British, their Hessian mercenaries, and the merciless winter weather. But he had another enemy that the history books ignore, an enemy that meant well but almost destroyed his army at Valley Forge. In Pennsylvania, where the main force of Washington's army was quartered ... the legislature ... decided to try a period of price control limited to those commodities needed for use by the army. ... The prices of uncontrolled goods, mostly imported, rose to record heights. Most farmers kept back their produce, refusing to sell at what they regarded as an unfair price. Some who had large families to take care of even secretly sold their food to the British who paid in gold. As a result, George Washington's army nearly starved to death.
~ William J. Baumol and Alan S. Blind, Economics Principles and Policy, Sixth Edition

When it comes to open combat, there is a universal strategy often adopted by military personnel — cutting off or damaging the supply channels. Whether the commodity is gasoline, weaponry, first aid supplies, or food, the lack of any one of these is enough to bring any army to its knees. Without these vital supplies, the army lacks the critical tools necessary to provide protection, repair and nourishment to its fighting units.

What if the supply lines that support the human body are cut off? Would the body be able to win the intense battles for survival raging within it each day? The answer is clearly no. Our cells are the supply lines that struggle each day to keep us healthy. Most people probably don't even realize the very important work our cells constantly perform inside the body. I (Kristy) will try to paint a mental picture for you.

Internally, the sixty trillion cells that make up your human frame are constantly on the march. They are duking it out with external invaders such as chemical toxins in the air you breathe, the water you drink, and the food you eat. Each day your cells must defend themselves against these dangerous attackers, while at the same time plotting a counterattack against bacteria and viruses that have slipped past the protective barriers and invaded your cellular city.

The war is a silent one; no gunshots or bombshells are heard. In fact, you can't even tell it is taking place. Nevertheless, destruction spreads rapidly and the body's cry for help is often ignored until symptoms of a chronic disease show up. Within the tissues and organs, white blood cells go to work on special assignments seeking, killing, and destroying these foreign invaders. This group of soldiers is the immune system. They have special names — T-lymphocytes, neutrophils, and macrophages. It is critical that this immune system battalion receive proper nourishment in order to fight.

But wait. There is a problem. The very food supply meant to feed this group has been attacked or destroyed by the enemy. The quality of fruit and vegetables, on which the immune system relies for strength, has been damaged. Vitamins, minerals, enzymes, and phytonutrients are missing from the food. The entire nutrient content has been sabotaged. Slowly, the army of immunity cells begins to succumb to the enemies within. How did this happen? How did the food God created to sustain our immune systems change so drastically? It's not a very pretty story. But here goes.

It started many years ago when farming went from being just a way to take care of individual families to a business venture based on mass production. With this undertaking, guidelines for proper crop rotation began to be ignored, thus depriving the soil of essential minerals needed for human health. Fruit and vegetables are picked "green" or before they are allowed to ripen on the vine, just to endure transport and make it to grocery store shelves without damage. By not allowing the fruit and vegetables to complete their vine-ripening process, farmers prevent us from receiving beneficial amounts of plant phytonutrients critical for disease prevention.

Simply allowing a banana or a tomato to ripen in a brown paper bag just does not do the trick. Even if we chose to be radical and consume a diet solely of fruit and vegetables to "be super healthy," we could never eat enough to provide all the required nutrients our internal army needs to protect and maintain our health. Let me paint the picture for you:

- In 1948, a cup of spinach contained 158 mg of iron per 100 grams
- In 1956, a cup of spinach contained 27 mg of iron per 100 grams
- In 1998, a cup of spinach contained about 2 mg of iron per 100 grams

Today, you would have to eat over seventy-five cups of spinach to get the same amount of nutrition available fifty-six years ago. Consuming this amount of food is virtually impossible. Even the five to nine servings of fruit and vegetables recommended by most nutritionists are outside the radar screen of most individuals. Who has the time or the capacity to eat that much food? No one. Therefore, our nation's health has been on a continual decline as a result of this nutrient deterioration in the fruit and vegetables now on the market.

But our early ancestors from the hunter-gatherer period of history had far better selections. They could choose from a wide variety of freshly picked food that was nutrient dense and required minimal or no processing to prepare. In fact, food was often eaten shortly after being picked or gathered. According to C. Leigh Broadhurst, Ph.D., author of the *The Evolutionary Diet*, hunter-gatherer meals consisted of small portions of lean meat (including game, reptiles, amphibians, and insects), fish, large amounts of raw fruit and vegetables, and occasional nuts and seeds. It is estimated they ate approximately three times the amount of vegetables and fruit eaten today. Grown in nutrient-dense soil, the food selections of the hunter-gatherers were high in vital nutrients such as phytochemicals, vitamins, and minerals. As a result, the people who lived during this time were taller, leaner, stronger, and healthier.

The people of this era also engaged in a great deal of physical activity as part of everyday life. They had no need for fitness centers and stationary weight equipment to maintain proper bone and muscle integrity because their daily chores of hunting, gathering, digging, and carrying heavy objects gave them a complete workout. In addition, the hunter-gatherers moved a lot from place to place to find food. So they *had* to be in good physical condition to stay alive. "The majority of our ancestors' activities (except sleeping) required more energy (and, therefore, more food) than our typical activities of today. For example, a 132-pound woman burns 720 calories of energy during eight hours of office work. In comparison, her ancestor burned 2,160 calories gathering food in the same amount of time." (Montoye HJ; Kemper HCG; Saris WHM; Washburn RA; *Measuring Physical Activity and Energy*. Champaign, Illinois: Human Kinetics, 1996).

Because of the high physical demands placed on their lifestyle, the hunter-gatherers had to eat extremely large amounts of food. They ate frequently and could do so without weight gain or the health conditions that plague us today, such as obesity and high blood pressure. Again, the secret to their superior state of health can be attributed to their lifestyle, including the types of food they ate and the amount of exercise they got.

When the hunter-gatherer era was replaced by an agriculturally-based society, people changed from a diet of high variety nutrients to a few food staples such as potatoes, rice, and wheat. Unfortunately, this loss in variety had a severe effect on the health of many, as it is impossible to reach optimal nutritional levels by consuming the same food products. Over time, people actually became shorter and weaker. And in America, our nation's health has been on a continual decline despite medical advances.

Now that we are a modernized society with high-tech kitchen gadgets there is yet another variable that affects the nutrient content of food, specifically fruit and vegetables. It is the post-harvesting practices that occur in our very own kitchens — storage, washing, chopping, boiling, microwaving, freezing, and canning. In *From the Farm to the Kitchen Table: A Review of the Nutrient Losses in Foods,* Jane Ramberg and Bill McAnalley, Ph.D., capture the effects of our modern day food practices. In essence, the modern-day conveniences of stoves, microwaves, refrigerators, and canned goods have taken us two steps backward on the path to nutritious eating.

- Green beans refrigerated after harvest lost more than 90 percent of their ascorbic acid (vitamin C) following sixteen days of refrigeration; broccoli lost about 50 percent of both their ascorbic acid and beta-carotene following five days of storage.
- When cooking, the water-soluble vitamins, particularly thiamine, vitamin C, and folate, are the most sensitive to heat. The amount of vitamin C lost during cooking depends on the degree of heat used.
- Food that is heated and then reheated, particularly if it is held for long periods over heat, suffers high losses of vitamin C, folate, and vitamin B6.
- Nutrient losses can be large when food is heated in water. When vegetables are boiled, many of the minerals are lost to the cooking water. Steaming and pressure-cooking are significantly better at retaining minerals than boiling. The most nutritious way to cook potatoes is to bake them unpeeled.
- Most losses of vitamin B in meat are due to prolonged storage and thawing.
- When compared with frozen vegetables, canned vegetables have twice fewer vitamin C, niacin, and riboflavin and over three times less thiamine.

So it is not enough just to purchase healthy food. You must also consider how to store and prepare the food in order to retain its vitamin and mineral nutrients. Canned vegetables are not your friends and microwaves are the body's worst enemy. Important nutrients such as vitamin C, which protects against cancer and viral and bacterial infections, or vitamin E, which aids in preventing blood clots, don't stand a chance when they are overcooked on the stove or fried with radiation in a microwave. It's better to buy fresh vegetables and steam them when you get home.

Physicians and nutritionists agree the changes in the Western diet over the last one hundred years are responsible for the increase in hypertension, diabetes, and some types of cancers. It has been known for centuries that the body needs a daily intake of specific nutrients from a variety of sources to stay healthy. Yet today this knowledge is blatantly ignored. Dr. Stephen Boyd noted in an article entitled "History of Nutrition and Health" that three major conditions can be alleviated with specific food nutrients:

Scurvy, a serious and often fatal disease causing hemorrhages of the gums, joints, and skin, was very common among those at sea for long periods. In 1753, it was discovered that consumption of citrus fruit, such as lemons and limes, not only cured scurvy but also prevented its recurrence. Henceforth, the British navy supplemented sailors' diets with limes and other citrus fruits and, consequently, British sailors became known as "Limeys." Two hundred years later the missing ingredient was identified as vitamin C.

Beriberi was another serious and often fatal disease affecting the nerves, muscles, and heart, first described in the fifteenth century and subsequently demonstrated in the nineteenth century to be a consequence of eating polished white rice. "Polishing" was the process of removing the outer brown layer of rice. The disease could be cured and prevented by eating brown unpolished rice and, as was shown experimentally, by adding the rice "polishings" back in the diet. In this case, the missing nutritional component was vitamin B1. It is interesting that the 1929 Nobel Prize for

Medicine was awarded for the discovery that dietary supplementation could correct this condition.

The third of the classic dietary deficiency diseases was pellagra, which caused cracking of the skin, diarrhea, dementia, and, in addition, death to 50 percent of those who suffered from it. In the nineteenth and early part of the twentieth centuries, pellagra was at epidemic levels in institutions such as asylums and orphanages. First thought to be an infectious disease caused by bacteria, it was conclusively demonstrated in 1918 that pellagra was caused by a deficiency resulting from a monotonous, largely corn-based diet. Supplementing the diet with wheat germ, fruit, and vegetables completely cured the disease and prevented recurrence.

In all of the above historical accounts, serious diseases were clearly documented to be associated not with an inadequate quantity of food but with an insufficiency of a dietary ingredient. Once this was understood, these diseases could be cured and prevented by appropriate dietary supplementation.

The concept of fortifying our bodies with dietary supplements has been a controversial topic for years, but their merits have finally been validated in conventional healthcare circles. After years and years of debate, there is widespread agreement among healthcare professionals that our standard food supply has been damaged to the extent that it is insufficient for providing essential nutrients and, therefore, external fortification is critical to sustaining life. In fact, this conclusion is now endorsed by the hallowed *Journal of the American Medical Association,* which recently reversed its earlier position on dietary supplements. In the June 19, 2002, issue, *JAMA* said, "Most people do not consume an optimal amount of all vitamins by diet alone. ... It appears prudent for all adults to take vitamin supplements."

Baby boomers have jumped on the supplement bandwagon. Members of this group have a lot of influence and a lot of reasons to fortify their bodies as they hit their sixties and healthcare gets more expensive. They've also come to realize the answer is not in pharmaceutical drugs. This same population that prompted personal computer and SUV sales is now declaring drugs are too toxic, too expensive, and too unreliable.

JAMA estimates 50 percent of all patients are now seeking more natural, alternative forms of healthcare. That being the case, many have begun to add dietary supplements to their diets. U.S. sales of dietary supplements totaled $17.1 billion in 2000 and the *Nutrition Business Journal* projects the market will hit $92 billion by 2030. Traditional health care professionals also endorse the use of this form of preventive nutrition. Seventy percent of practicing physicians are recommending dietary supplements (*Drug Topics*, June 2001) and pharmacists are now endorsing the benefits of supplements.

With the benefits of supplements recognized by healthcare professionals and public demands for more information and non-toxic healthcare options, Congress in 1994 passed the Dietary Supplement Health Education Act (DSHEA). By passing this statute, our lawmakers agreed a preventive approach to health and wellness was long overdue and included the following declaration in the DSHEA text:

1. The importance of nutrition and the benefits of dietary supplements to health promotion and disease prevention have been documented increasingly in scientific studies.
2. There is a link between the ingestion of certain nutrients or dietary supplements and the prevention of chronic diseases such as cancer, heart disease, and osteoporosis.
3. Preventive health measures, including education, good nutrition, and appropriate use of safe nutritional supplements, will limit the incidence of chronic diseases and reduce long-term health care expenditures.

So there you have it. Even Congress agrees it is necessary to take additional nutrients to replace those that may be missing from the food we buy at the grocery store. While the choices of supplementation are many, it is important we understand that our bodies were designed to accept and function from the supply of nutrients found in food; therefore, it is only natural that we supplement with *food-based* supplements, and not synthetic chemical vitamins and pills. In *How to Survive on a Toxic Planet*, Dr. Steve Nugent identifies seven categories of supplements deemed critical for support of the body's various systems.

1. Essential vitamins and minerals to create healthy cells and facilitate internal reactions

2. Glyconutrients for cellular communication and proper immune system function
3. Antioxidants to protect cells from oxidative damage
4. Phytonutrients (plant nutrients) to detoxify the body system
5. Phytohormones (plant hormones) for proper function of glands and the hormonal system
6. Essential fatty acids (omega 3 and omega 6 fats) for cellular regeneration and hormonal system function
7. Essential amino acids for building protein

Without these additional nutrients, your cellular city is left unguarded and internal enemies can take over. Consult a natural health care professional for specific products.

I (Kristy) remember when I was first informed that if I wanted truly to prevent disease, I had to start taking supplements daily. This lecture came from the same doctor brother-in-law who challenged me to change my diet. The mere thought of having to swallow all of those pills — some big, some small — on a daily basis just made me sick to my stomach. (Probably because I knew I would have a very hard time getting them down!)

However, my brother-in-law put it to me in a different way. He asked, "Kristy, don't you pay your house insurance every month?"

"Yes," I answered.

"Don't you pay your car insurance every month?"

"Yes."

"Then what are you doing to provide *health assurance* every month?" He then explained supplements are a necessary part of my preventive health assurance plan and there was no way around it.

I knew he was dropping some heavy knowledge on me and I had no choice but to listen, revise my monthly budget to include supplements, and obey. Besides, he is a trained and skilled holistic doctor and I am not. I was reminded of the Scripture in Proverbs: "Apply your heart to instruction, and your ears to words of knowledge" (Proverbs 23:12). I realized his words of wisdom were provided out of love and were meant for my protection.

Thomas Edison once said, "The doctor of the future will give no medicines, but will interest his patients in the care of the human frame, in diet, and in the causes of disease." We could all learn from this legendary inventor. It is only when we take interest and show concern for what is going on inside the body on a cellular level that we can truly reign over the temptation to feed our cells nutritionally bankrupt food *and* take preventive steps to provide additional nourishment. So decide now to restock all of your supplies in this battle for health. Get nutritional reinforcements in the form of vitamins, minerals, antioxidants, phytonutrients, and glyconutrients. They can replenish what the enemy has stolen from the contents of your grocery store bags.

Chapter Summary

1. Our food supply system has been robbed over the years of essential nutrients due to changes in farming practices and food preparation techniques.
2. It is important to include nutritional supplements as a part of an optimal health plan because today's food does not contain enough of what we need.
3. Healthcare professionals and Congress have recognized the need for dietary supplements and endorsed them as part of a healthy lifestyle regimen.
4. Categories of nutritional supplements deemed critical for the body include: vitamins & minerals, glyconutrients, antioxidants, phytonutrients, phytohormones, essential fatty acids, and essential amino acids.

Chapter Twenty

Faith Without Works

So also faith, if it does not have works (deeds and actions of obedience to back it up), by itself is destitute of power (inoperative, dead). ~ James 2:17 (AMP)

Imagine this scenario: It is Sunday morning and you arrive at church late, but you manage to make it to your favorite seat along the aisle and just behind the camera crew that tapes the service for television. You are thankful you did not miss praise and worship because that is the part of service that wakes you up and gives you a sense of peace after your hour-long commute to the church. As the choir gracefully releases their last harmonized note of the song "Jehovah Jireh," you feel you are now in a state of mind to receive the Word about to come forth. You are excited because today's sermon is a continuation of the series "Possessing My Harvest." Today, your pastor is going to unleash the keys to acquiring all of the material blessings you desire. You've got your red pen and your yellow highlighter in hand, and you are ready to go.

Quickly, the pastor takes you to Deuteronomy 8:18. "But thou shalt remember the Lord thy God: for it is he that giveth thee power to get wealth, that he may establish his covenant which he sware unto thy fathers, as it is this day" (KJV). Following Deuteronomy, you are lead to 2 Chronicles 20:20, which reads in part, "Believe in the Lord your God, so shall ye be established; believe his prophets, so shall ye prosper" (KJV). Next, you are asked to turn to Job 36:11. "If they obey and serve him, they shall spend their days in prosperity, and their years in pleasures" (KJV). Last, he concludes the sermon with a word of wisdom from Proverbs. "The blessing of the Lord, it maketh rich, and he addeth no sorrow with it." (Proverbs 10:22 KJV). (Proverbs 13:22 KJV).

Once again, you are encouraged by the message for the day, for you are confident you have learned how to move away from the world's economic system and receive the harvest God has designed for you. You are prepared to leave for home with a warm, fuzzy feeling inside, knowing that "increase" is yours and your days of walking in prosperity are coming soon. You can almost touch the new black BMW you plan to purchase, and envision the colors you'll select to paint the walls of that new five-bedroom house you want.

Suddenly, before you are released from the sanctuary, the order of service takes a twist. The pastor announces he is led to have a healing service and begins to call to the altar those in the congregation who need to be healed. You take a quick glance at your watch and see the service is supposed to end in approximately fifteen minutes. Knowing you have a lunch appointment at the local pancake house after church, you are slightly concerned things may run longer than expected now that the healing program has begun. Realizing there is nothing you can do, you reposition yourself in your seat and wait for what you expect to be a fifteen-minute healing service.

Heeding the pastor's altar call, one by one individuals from all sections of the sanctuary head to the front of the room. You begin counting them, for you know the number of people approaching the pastor will impact whether you make it to lunch on time. You mumble softly to yourself, "Ten ... twenty-five ... fifty ... seventy-five ... 125."

At this point you lose count and begin to estimate the number of people who have surrounded the pastor. You assume there are about 250 people at the front of the room, and more people are leaving their chairs and are making a beeline to the altar. You then estimate 350 people ... 400 ... 425. At this point you are speechless. You had no idea so many people were suffering with sickness! You resolve to forget about your lunch date, because the healing service you thought would take fifteen minutes is destined to last a few hours.

Have you ever experienced a situation like this? Over eight years ago I (Kristy) attended my very first healing service and found it to be quite disturbing because it happened just as I've described. At the time, I just stood back and watched in awe as massive numbers of people headed to the altar. After a while I had to stop praying because I was so overwhelmed by the number of people going forward as well as the various health problems they shared that I just fell back into my chair and began to cry. I can remember saying to the Lord, "Father, you did not tell me this many Christians were sick!" How could this be? Eventually, there were more people at the altar than the number who remained seated. As a new Christian at the time, I was shocked.

How could there be more sick people in the congregation than healthy people? How had Satan been allowed to infiltrate the church, attack such a large number of people and hold them captive? It was a Sunday with sharp contrasts. While the sermon focused on prosperity, the healing service exposed an enormous amount of "poverty" in the church. All too often, believers are single minded when it comes to prosperity. They usually think being prosperous is only about having material possessions. But having all the silver and gold is only part of the story. God wants us to prosper in all areas of our lives.

Prosperity means having peace, joy, godly relationships, money, land, houses, cars, family members who have accepted Christ, and a whole host of other things including good health. What good is it to be financially fit and not physically fit? What good is it to be debt free and have a bank account full of money, and be laid up in the hospital, unable to move physically to place the money in the hands of the people or organizations that could benefit from your donation? Thus, your ability to use wealth is conditional. That condition is you must be around long enough to spend it. Imagine that! The opportunity to use your financial wealth to do the things you desire depends on how healthy you are.

God makes this clear in 3 John 2: "Beloved, I wish above all things that thou mayest prosper and be in health, even as thy soul prospereth" (KJV). How do we get health prosperity? It all starts with knowing God's plan for your life. How do you know his plan? By studying the Word of God. Once you know God's plan as laid out in the bible, how do you begin applying it to your life? By developing an image of that plan in your mind. How do you do that? By meditating on God's Word through reading it, pondering it, speaking it, and ultimately believing it.

Meditating on God's Word is a process of feeding your mind, will, emotions, intellect, and conscious — which make up the soul — with the truth about how we should really live. In other words, meditating on God's Word renews your mind to think the way God wants you to think instead of how the world wants you to think. Everything around us tells us it's normal to be sick and on medication, that it's normal to always be in need, and that it's normal to only look for answers in doctors and surgery. But the bible enlightens us on how to live God's way, the supernatural way in which we were originally built to live.

There is a lot of talk these days in the body of Christ about a coming "wealth transfer." Proverbs 13:22 is one of the Scriptures cited in support of this transfer: "A good man leaveth an inheritance to his children's children: and the wealth of the sinner is laid up for the just" (KJV). Psalm 105:44 is another favorite: "And (he) gave them the lands of the heathen: and they inherited the labour of the people" (KJV). What does this mean in many church circles? That the wealth of those who do not accept Jesus as Lord and Savior will end up in the hands of Christians. Yes, children of God need wealth and resources to exercise dominion over the earth as God directed, but it takes more than money to do that. It also takes good health.

Webster's Dictionary defines "transfer" as: "To move to a different place, region, or situation; to take over the possession or control of; a conveyance of right, title, or interest in real or personal property from one person to another." Meditate on this definition because it describes what God wants us to have in terms of wealth *and* health. The first phrase makes reference to moving from one place to another — i.e., moving from State A to State B. One also could move from Condition A to Condition B. To make it even plainer, one could move from having diabetes to not having diabetes. In all cases, movement or action is required. This means we have to do something. Faith without works is dead. What type of action is required? Depending on the situation and God's direction, God may suggest any of the following:

- Daily meditation on healing scriptures
- Separation from negative elements
- Fasting and praying
- Surgery or other intervention by a medical doctor
- Seeking out the assistance of holistic health practitioners — chiropractors, nutritionists, naturopaths
- Changing your diet
- Beginning an exercise program

Recognize God has a specific way of healing that is unique to each individual. You cannot necessarily predict the exact method he has selected for you based on what he did for another person. Every individual is different and God's plan of action will differ from person to person. It is important that you spend time with God and ask for his direction. It is through the guidance of the Holy Spirit that you will receive your marching orders. And I do mean marching orders! Just as a marine is given his assignment and proceeds to fulfill his assignment quickly, diligently, and with no questions asked, when God gives you a plan of action to better your health you must follow that plan with complete compliance.

The second phrase in the definition of "transfer" speaks of taking control. In terms of your health, optimal health must be taken or seized. "And from the days of John the Baptist until now the kingdom of heaven suffereth violence, and the violent take it by force" (Matthew 11:12 KJV). If you are fighting with a health challenge but your desire is to walk in divine health, then it is necessary for you to take control of the situation. Again, taking control requires *action*. When a leader takes control of a board meeting or when a commander takes control of an army, he exercises his authority.

Walking in the fullness of the authority God has given us is a choice. Each and every day, you have a choice whether you are going to lie in bed or go downstairs and speed-walk a couple of miles on your treadmill. You have a choice whether you are going to fix sausage, pancakes, and coffee for breakfast, or pull an apple and a pear from your untouched fruit bowl sitting in the middle of your kitchen table. The choice is yours.

This leads us to the third part of the definition for "transfer": "a conveyance of right, title, or interest in real or personal property from one person to another." God has given us the right to be healthy. This was God's plan for us from the very beginning. Divine health is the ultimate representation of our status as God's children. The following passages confirm this is God's desire for his children:

> **For I will restore health unto thee, and I will heal thee of thy wounds, saith the Lord; because they called thee an Outcast, saying, This is Zion, whom no man seeketh after.**
> **~ *Jeremiah 30:17 (KJV)***

> **Bless the Lord, O my soul, and forget not all his benefits: Who forgiveth all thine iniquities; who healeth all thy diseases. ~ *Psalm 103:2-3 (KJV)***

"Restore" is a key word in the Jeremiah scripture cited above. God's original blueprint for our bodies was not defective. Sickness and disease were never supposed to exist. There was no cancer gene in Adam and Eve when God created the first family. The opportunity for it to crop up in our bodies came with the fall of man. But Jesus took care of all this on the cross. His sacrifice restored the right to divine health which is a wonderful condition where sickness and disease cannot touch us.

Unfortunately, far too many believers in Christ continue to accept sickness as a form of punishment merely because they do not fully understand the gift of health freely given to them through Jesus' birth and death. The health benefits package we received through the crucifixion is detailed in the book of Isaiah. It is a preview of what later occurred on the cross:

> **He was despised and rejected and forsaken by men, a Man of sorrows and pains, and acquainted with grief and sickness; and like One from Whom men hide their faces He was despised, and we did not appreciate His worth or have**

any esteem for Him. Surely He has borne our griefs (sicknesses, weaknesses, and distresses) and carried our sorrows and pains [of punishment], yet we [ignorantly] considered Him stricken, smitten, and afflicted by God [as if with leprosy]. But He was wounded for our transgressions, He was bruised for our guilt and iniquities; the chastisement [needful to obtain] peace and well-being for us was upon Him, and with the stripes [that wounded] Him we are healed and made whole. ~ Isaiah 53:3-5 (AMP)

Even before he was nailed to the cross, Jesus endured the punishment for what his religious opponents thought was heresy. They considered his teachings contrary to those of the Jewish faith. At that time, the punishment for heresy was a sentence to the whipping post where the accused received thirty-nine stripes across the back. The stripes were applied to Jesus' bare back with a leather whip that contained bits of steel, copper, and brass. Upon impact with his flesh, blood immediately flowed. His enduring this first stage of punishment has a direct correlation to the level of health we are guaranteed today. Evangelist R.W. Schambach describes it this way in his book *4 Lambs*: "Medical science says there are thirty-nine original sicknesses, and from those original thirty-nine there are hundreds, maybe even thousands, of sicknesses and diseases. But they all stem from the original thirty-nine. If that is true, then Jesus carried thirty-nine stripes on his back. I submit to you that Jesus carried a stripe for every sickness and disease you are carrying. If he carried it, you don't have any business carrying it, for by his stripes you are healed." Through the shedding of his own blood, Jesus became the sacrificial lamb upon the altar so we do not have to live with sickness and disease today. We have been redeemed from these curses.

The point to be made here is that one must fully understand and accept all that took place on the cross. Jesus accomplished everything at Calvary that needed to be done for us to be healed. If you can comprehend that it is unacceptable by God's standards that you surrender to a life with obesity, diabetes, or even cancer, then you are positioned to take hold of the next requirement to receive diving healing: believing. To believe you can receive healing requires that you have faith. Hebrews 11:1 defines faith as "the substance of things hoped for, the evidence of things not seen" (KJV). One must first believe in order to receive. When it comes to receiving our healing, the level of faith we have could impact how quickly the evidence of healing shows up.

The Bible contains several stories about how a person's faith resulted in immediate healing. Back then, thousands of people often flocked to Jesus' healing message. Many believed it, received it, and walked away well and whole. But they took action — sometimes bold action — to get their healing.

> *And behold, a leper came and worshiped Him, saying, "Lord, if You are willing, You can make me clean." Then Jesus put out His hand and touched him, saying "I am willing; be cleansed." Immediately his leprosy was cleansed.*
> *~ Matthew 8:2-3*

Lepers were social outcasts due to the contagiousness of their disease. They were sent off to colonies with others who were in the same condition and told not to mingle with the non-infected. So for this leper to even approach Jesus meant he first changed his mind about how he saw his life and then did something about it. The same is true for the woman with the issue of blood (mentioned in Chapter 12 of this book), who pressed through the crowd to touch the hem of Jesus' garment for her healing. And one of the most famous biblical accounts of someone getting healed at all costs is recorded in the book of Mark.

Jesus was ministering in a house in the city of Capernaum. The event should have been classified as "standing room only" because so many people had come out to see him. The house was full and there was even a large crowd that had formed a barricade around the front door. One man who was sick with palsy and on a stretcher was so determined to receive his healing that he solicited the assistance of four friends and committed an act of vandalism in order to get close to Jesus.

> *And when they could not get him to a place in front of Jesus because of the throng, they dug through the roof above Him; and when they had scooped out an opening, they let down the [thickly padded] quilt or mat upon which the paralyzed man lay. And when Jesus saw their faith [their confidence in God through Him], He said to the paralyzed many, Son, your sins are forgiven [you] and put away [that is, the penalty is remitted, the sense of guilt removed, and you are made upright and in right standing with God]. And*

> *he arose at once and picked up the sleeping pad or mat and went out before them all, so that they were all amazed and recognized and praised and thanked God, saying, We have never seen anything like this before!*
> ~ *Mark 2:4-5, 12 (AMP)*

In this case, not only did the sickly man have a high level of faith, his faith was matched by that of his four daring friends! They were all so confident that healing would occur that they broke with all proper protocol to join the healing service by tearing through the roof of someone's house! As a result, Jesus honored their faith and their courageous act.

Another incident where faith is exercised is depicted when Jesus and his disciples were leaving Jericho and a blind beggar, Bartimaeus, caught wind that Jesus of Nazareth was about to pass by. Wanting to seize hold of his healing, Bartimaeus took action.

> *And when he heard that is was Jesus of Nazareth, he began to shout, saying, Jesus, Son of David, have pity and mercy on me (now)! And many severely censured and reproved him, telling him to keep still but he kept on shouting out all the more, You Son of David, have pity and mercy on me (now)! And Jesus stopped and said, Call him. And they called the blind man, telling him, Take courage! Get up! He is calling you. And throwing off his outer garment, he leaped up and came to Jesus. And Jesus said to him, What do you want Me to do for you? And the blind man said to Him, Master, let me receive my sight. And Jesus said to him, Go your way; your faith has healed you. And at once he received his sight and accompanied Jesus on the road.*
> ~ *Mark 10:47-52 (AMP)*

Despite the crowd's efforts to quiet him, Bartimaeus pressed on and got his healing. He demonstrated mastery of the equation for divine healing. He understood the significance of Jesus being in town, believed he would heal him, acted on that faith and immediately received his sight. He did not have to wait months or years; his health transfer was sudden.

One must understand there is a difference between divine healing and divine health. Let's begin with an explanation of divine healing. God has the power to heal any condition. This is why we can witness a man in a wheelchair receive the ability to walk in less than five minutes, after the power of God flows through his body. What occurred is "divine healing," which is a sudden event. Sometimes the manifestation or evidence of healing may be instantaneous or it may occur over a period of time. It may take several minutes, hours, days, weeks, or years to visually see the results of God's healing hand; only God controls the time clock. Isaiah 55:8-9 reminds us of God's way of operating: "My thoughts are not your thoughts, nor are your ways My ways." He operates at a much higher level than our feeble minds are capable of understanding. But regardless of when divine healing manifests, God is the initiator and is to be given full credit for the result.

Now, let's take a look at the concept of divine health. Divine health is not the same as divine healing. If one needs healing, then it can be inferred he or she is sick. But if one has health, then it means he or she is "staying well." Referring back to the healing service described at the beginning of this chapter, just because someone stood in line, got "hands laid" on him or her, and received a healing does not mean he or she will walk in divine health going forward.

Divine health is related to maintenance. Unlike divine healing, it is a process and not a single event. It is the result of living a lifestyle of daily practices that promote optimal health. These practices may include eating healthy, exercising daily, and reducing stress factors. Hence, when God does the miracle of healing in us, the least we can do is stand firm and be good stewards over his handiwork. What parents would not be appalled to give their teenager a brand-new car only to find it full of junk with no oil in the engine six months later? Perhaps many of us look like that teenager to God when it comes to our physical maintenance. The world not only needs to see that God is faithful to bless us, but also that we are faithful to preserve his blessing in all areas of our lives.

I (Kristy) once witnessed a woman who had received healing from cancer during a church service. However, after receiving healing she left church, went straight to the grocery store, and bought a large bag of potato chips, which she began to eat immediately. Does this sound logical? Better yet, does this sound faithful? This woman fell back into the same lifestyle trap that may have contributed to her cancer condition in the first place. Yes, she received healing, but she did not follow with a corresponding action to fiercely pursue, obtain, and maintain a condition of divine health. God wants us to do our part to keep the healing he gives us. It is during this post-healing period when the person healed must take focused, consistent action to stay healed.

Although Satan might open the door to countless ways for us to destroy our health, we are the ones who decide whether or not to walk through that door. Oftentimes, if we just look in the mirror, we will see our own worst enemy when it comes to walking in divine health. That person staring back at us is the one who self-inflicts bodily injury day after day with ice cream, cake, hamburgers, lunchmeat, cheese, pizza, sodas, etc. It is time that we all put on our soldier's gear, stop shooting ourselves with these dietary bullets, and start taking aim at habits and behaviors that destroy our health. God has given us the authority to do this. When we start using our authority, we will begin to see the health transfer take place one person at a time, church by church, city by city, and nation by nation.

Earnest believers try hard every day to live how God wants them to live. They realize the benefits of obeying their heavenly Father. Let's extend this awareness to the very important area of health and nutrition. Obedience paves the way to blessings. Disobedience invites disease. Romans 12:1-2 says, "I beseech you therefore, brethren, by the mercies of God, that ye present your bodies a living sacrifice, holy, acceptable unto God, which is your reasonable service. And be not conformed to this world: but be ye transformed by the renewing of your mind, that ye may prove what is that good, and acceptable, and perfect will of God."

Here, God is loudly requesting that we not conform to the world's way of living. The body of Christ has separated itself from the world when it comes to the outer trappings of Christian life. Many of us changed the way we dressed after we got saved. We changed the way we talk — stopped cursing and started talking "Christianese." The music from our old juke joint days went in the trash and was replaced with Shirley Caesar, the Brooklyn Tabernacle Choir, or the Gaithers. Some of us stopped gambling, smoking, drinking, and doing anything else we were told Christians did not do. But we failed to change the way we eat, resulting in a neglect of our inner temple. We kept on eating junk and not exercising regularly. As a result, we are now part of the world's healthcare crisis instead of being examples of the solution. Is this the image we want to project as God's elect? As the Apostle Paul would say, "God forbid!"

In Exodus, God made a strong declaration to the ancient Hebrews from which we could benefit if we followed suit: "If thou wilt diligently hearken to the voice of the Lord thy God, and wilt do that which is right in his sight, and wilt give ear to his commandments, and keep all his statutes, I will put none of the diseases upon thee, which I have brought upon the Egyptians: for I am the Lord that healeth thee" (Exodus 15:26 KJV). God tells us if we hear and do what he tells us to do, even in the area of eating, we can overcome the healthcare crisis and receive the blessing of divine health. Yet, please understand, action is first required on our part.

Chapter Summary

1. God is a healer.
2. Divine healing is an event.
3. Divine health means staying well.
4. Attaining and maintaining health and healing require a continual effort on our part.

Chapter Twenty-One

Amazing Grace

Amazing Grace, how sweet the sound, that saved a wretch like me.
I once was lost but now am found, was blind, but now, I see.

T'was Grace that taught my heart to fear, and Grace, my fears relieved.
How precious did that Grace appear, the hour I first believed.
- **John Newton (1725 – 1807)**

Amazing Grace is a song about salvation. Former slave trader John Newton, who cried out to God during a horrific storm while at sea, wrote it. Accrediting his safety to the power and grace of God, Newton became a Christian and eventually a priest in the Church of England. Many years later, he wrote the words above to use with his congregation.

I (Kristy) was challenged to get a grip on my health in 1997. I was thirty years old at the time. Still occupationally married to the processed food industry, my kitchen cabinets and refrigerator were a reflection of my level of commitment. Processed cereal, Pop-Tarts, bagels, cookies, microwave meals, microwave popcorn, microwave pizza, yogurt, 2 percent milk, and, of course, my all-time favorite: ice cream, were included. I had all the components of what I thought should be food heaven at the time. However, I was also quite sickly.

Weekly bouts of constipation and indigestion were normal for me. And fatigue? I was exhausted every day. After my hour commute home from work, I would routinely pass out on my couch within fifteen minutes of arrival. But that was only after I ate my Wendy's chicken sandwich and chocolate Frosty. I always would manage to wake up around eleven p.m., do a bit of paperwork, and then return to sleep until morning.

My chain got yanked when my brother-in-law, a chiropractor and nutritionist, visited me from out-of-state and observed my pitiful routine. Concerned with the amount of sleep I required to function, he felt the need to confront me. He asked, "Kristy, do you know why you are so tired all the time?" The best answer I could find was, "Work."

Unfortunately, that was not the correct answer. He then escorted me into my kitchen and started opening my cabinets and propped open my refrigerator. Then he shed quite a bit of light on my state of health. "Kristy, you have a hormonal imbalance and are tired because of the way you eat! If you continue to eat all this garbage you maintain in this house, you WILL have a disease by the time you hit age forty-five! Diabetes, high blood pressure, high cholesterol — pick one."

Wow! I was speechless and humbled at the same time. I stood numb as he pointed at all of my precious commodities and commanded they be absent from my kitchen the next time he came to visit. Not only did he challenge me, he also took a direct swipe at the very industry I had faithfully served for so many years. I knew his lecture was not meant to offend me, but to bring correction. It was actually a sermon meant to save my life. So, I made the decision to listen and obey. That passage in Proverbs 23:12 came to mind again: "Apply your heart to instruction, and your ears to words of knowledge."

There was not a word I could say in my defense other than ask, "What should I do?" His response saved my life. He said, "Clean out these cabinets and start reading about nutrition." I heeded his advice the very next week. Books, videos, audiotapes, and seminars — if it was about nutrition, I absorbed myself in it. The more I read, the more I realized I was at fault. By not caring for my temple, I was disobeying God. Through ignorance, I had fed my body so poorly that over the long-term, a stage had been set where disease could come in and destroy me.

My transition to a healthier lifestyle was not without bumps and bruises. I allowed myself a year to make the change. One month I removed microwave meals, the next month it was ice cream. Bit by bit I learned healthier substitutes to consume. I noticed the more I pursued optimal health and nutrition, the more God led me to the resources that could help me. Grace prevailed, and to this day my life has never been the same.

I (Christine) had a rude awakening about food one Mother's Day weekend. We call these events "revelations" in the body of Christ. I had been eating very badly for about a year — just grabbing whatever I could because I worked such long hours. I also had been battling insomnia for weeks. Well, that weekend I was rushing around like a chicken with its head cut off. I was running late for a flight but was trying to get some things finished for my mom. So instead of eating a normal breakfast, I grabbed a piece of pound cake she had baked. I then sped off to the airport.

By the time I arrived at the airport, I realized I did not feel well and was hungry for some "real food." So I stopped at a fast-food restaurant and grabbed some fried chicken and French fries. I topped off the meal with some apple pie, raced to drop off the rental car, and ran to my terminal gate with my carry-on luggage in tow. I felt a little woozy, but thought it was due to my hectic pace.

By the time my flight was fully airborne, I was as sick as a dog. I broke out in a cold sweat. My hands were shaking. I was quite nauseous and searched my seatback for the little baggie I thought I'd never have to use on an airplane. I felt like crying but did not want to draw attention to myself. Thankfully, I had the entire row to myself. A flight attendant noticed my sickly look and asked in a grave voice, "Are you all right?" I said, "I will be as soon as this flight is over."

That hour-and-fifteen-minute trip from Memphis to Chicago seemed like a transatlantic journey. All the while I prayed, "Lord, if you let me off this flight without an episode that will embarrass me, I promise you I will take better care of my body!" Well, he did and I did. I went home and got down on my knees in prayer. I repented for being a bad steward over my body. I asked the Lord to show me how to eat properly and take control of my cravings for sweets and other unhealthy foods. I asked him to help me fast and learn how to live a fasted life — how not to let my body tell me what to do.

For two-and-a-half days, I ate nothing. I only drank water. By the end of the second day, I felt wonderful! My digestive problems were gone. I could sleep through the night. My thoughts cleared up! I felt like a new person. I had not realized how miserable I had been. I then sat down and devised a meal plan that worked for me. I basically cut out everything except vegetables. I later added some occasional eggs, fish, and poultry (free-range, and antibiotic- and hormone-free).

I had actually implemented a semi-detoxification plan, although I did not know it at the time. I followed this regimen for thirty days to discipline my body and tacked on another five days for good measure. I was so happy and feeling so well, I did not want to mess up anything. The difference was mind-boggling. I was still sleeping through the night and could actually get through the day without throwing up and embarrassing myself.

During that thirty-five-day period, I had no cravings for sugar or other junk food. I ate three wholesome meals a day regardless of my schedule. I brown-bagged my lunch every day. I even went on business trips with my own food and, yes, I walked right into meetings (even with VIPs) with my own food. I avoided restaurants whenever possible.

When this was unavoidable, I special ordered my food. I became more consistent with my exercise routine. I prayed. I thanked God. Then I preached this lifestyle change to anyone who would listen. I was mocked, challenged, and applauded. But it did not matter what anyone else thought. God understood and continued to bless my efforts.

While you may not be able to relate to our personal dietary turning points, perhaps you can identify with at least one or more people or situations mentioned elsewhere in this book. For some of you, reading about the lady who felt surrounded by the enemy at work and at home may have made you scream, "That's me!" For others, you may have seen yourself as one of the four hundred people in the church service healing line as described in Chapter 20, and are still faithfully believing God to be made whole. Regardless of the circumstances, one common thread exists: we all share a continuous struggle with food and physical inactivity that can adversely impact our health. No one is exempt.

Whether you hated vegetables growing up or became addicted to fast food and soft drinks in your teenage years, food is the big issue. For some of you, food problems are still lingering like a cobweb in the corner of the attic that just needs to be swept away. For others, you may recognize vital organs such as your thyroid, pancreas, or gallbladder are breaking down and you could stand to shed forty pounds or more. Or, you may be suffering from aches and pains or poor digestion, or just quite simply have lost your "get up and go."

Now that your food choices have been identified as the potential source of your ailments, your concern right now might be, "Is it really possible for me to make a successful change?" You may be thinking, "I have tried and failed at every diet under the sun and I am presently paying for a membership at a fitness club to which I never go, so how can I possibly succeed in making a permanent lifestyle change this time? I continue to fail time and time again, so why try now?"

After years of consulting with numerous clients (women in particular), I (Kristy) have heard these weary voices of concern and empathize with you wholeheartedly. I understand many of you may be hiding behind a veil of failure and shame, too frustrated to even want to put forth the effort to get healthy. In the past, you've tried to follow that diet plan perfectly every day without deviation. Things were going well until you went to that birthday party and had one tiny piece of pizza and a slice of chocolate cake topped with ice cream. After that, guilt set in. Guilt was followed by failure, and failure was followed by condemnation (feeling unworthy). Condemnation led to the end of your diet.

Understand that when you make mistakes, it is only natural to be bombarded by feelings of failure and remorse. However, you don't have to let these momentary lapses overtake you to the point of becoming paralyzed. Grace can prevail. And what exactly is grace? It is the bridge to God that we travel by faith. In short, grace can be described as "God's unmerited favor." It is kind of like divine assistance, help, or aid given to us from God, whether we feel we deserve it or not. Oftentimes, grace comes even without our asking. Grace reminds us we are not perfect creatures and only God is perfect. Grace is that something that gives us room to fail and yet recover from our failures without severe wounds. While we may stumble and fall routinely, grace allows us to get up and hold our heads high and try again. In essence, grace is what truly gives us freedom to fail. Without that freedom, most of us would be resistant to step out of our comfort zones and try new things.

Is it possible to receive God's grace even when it comes to eating poorly and mistreating your body? Absolutely! God's grace prevailed for me (Kristy) when he sent my brother-in-law to curtail my spree of microwave dining, possibly preventing a future disease down the road. Grace also prevailed for me (Christine) when I survived my airplane adventure without spilling my guts, but rather was allowed to return home safely and change my ways. Neither of us could have made these drastic changes without help from above. But rather, it was God's intervention that allowed us to see where we had failed (or sinned), enabled us to realize that "to err is human", and led us in the right direction so we could change successfully without continual guilt or condemnation. How wonderful grace is!

Whether you are a spiritual fanatic or one who has no concept of God, he is still watching over you and cares for your safety. The reason you are still alive after years of poor eating is solely due to his grace. Think about it. God could have allowed Satan to steal your life after eating one short-stack with bacon and sausage and a never-ending cup of coffee. Instead, he has provided a covering and has given you time to make health corrections before the fatty foods clog your arteries completely and it becomes too late. That's grace. It is solely through God's grace that we are able to make attempts at healthy eating, some of which may not be successful. God says to us, "I commend you for trying. Now get back on the wagon." That's how amazing God is. His grace is sufficient to help you overcome anything.

The benefits of walking in the freedom of this grace are available for everyone. But to truly be able to fully understand and receive His grace, you must first know who He is. If you are not in partnership with God, embarking upon a relationship with him is really quite simple. In fact, just one year prior to changing my diet and beginning a new way of eating, I (Kristy) also began a new relationship with my heavenly Father. Before then, I, too, did not fully understand this "God thing" and had no clue as to what church was all about or why so many people chose to wear crosses on chains around their necks. What I did know was Christmas was supposedly celebrated for a reason and someone had to have created the earth and the sun. In my mind, it could not have been man. Thus, my quest to find God began. And believe it or not, I did not have to hunt long. God's only requirement was that I ask for him to show himself to me. You can do the same. In your quiet time, you might whisper something as simple as this to him:

> Dear Lord, I admit I don't know who you are, but I long to learn more about you and your ways. Forgive me for following my own way and thinking I can make it on my own in this world without your heavenly guidance. I accept Jesus Christ as my Lord and Savior. I believe Jesus is the son of God who died to take away all the sins of the world, including mine. I ask and welcome him to come into my life and change me. I thank you, Lord, for your great sacrifice, for forgiving my sins, and for making me a part of the family of God.

A simple prayer between you and God. That's all it takes. Trust me. God will hear you and will respond beyond measure in your life. Now, if you want to be set apart or sanctified in your body, you might take it one step further and pray something like this:

> Dear Father, forgive me for not being a good steward over my physical temple, which you have given me for your service. I repent for repeatedly falling prey to food temptations. Help me to flee them. Thank you for your Word that has shown me the light on this very important subject. I reject food as my false god. I reject the lust of the eyes. I reject all traditions that cater to my fleshly dietary weaknesses that rob me of good health. I trust you to teach me how, when, and what to eat. I declare I am whole in spirit, soul, and body, and my flesh is subject to my spirit and will obey you in all things. I am adopting a healthy lifestyle so I may serve you and fulfill my divine calling. I will guard your temple like a good soldier. Thank you, Lord, for guiding my steps in this area as my heart plans its way. In the name of Jesus, my Lord and Savior, Amen.

So think about Thanksgivings when you ate until your stomach hurt, and Christmases when you gained an additional ten pounds and swore you'd join a health club in the New Year to work off the damage done to your body. God's grace has forgiven you of these "food sins," therefore it is high time you forgive yourself. The funny thing is, God actually granted you forgiveness long before you did anything wrong. That's how phenomenal God is. And when were you forgiven? At the very moment Jesus Christ was crucified on the cross, his blood disposed of your mistakes — past, present, and future. It is the blood of Jesus that God sees as atonement for our bodily neglect and allows forgiveness to occur. All you have to do is receive this wonderful gift, and you are declared righteous with God and in "good standing." In other words, God says, "You're okay. Everything is going to be all right."

> *For all have sinned and fall short of the glory of God, being justified freely by His grace through the redemption that is in Christ Jesus. ~ Romans 3:23-24*

> *Blessed and happy and to be envied is the person of whose sin the Lord will take no account nor reckon it against him. ~ Romans 4:8 (AMP)*

In addition, since we are crucified with Christ, our old man or nature was crucified with him. Sounds a bit churchy, but here's the ultimate result of Jesus' death. If you are known to have poor eating habits that have led to excessive weight gain and/or sickness, then that person died on the cross. If eating meat is your stronghold and your doctor has confirmed that eating too much of it is damaging your heart and arteries, then that meat-addicted person died on the cross. The person you hate to look at in the mirror every morning as you dress died on the cross.

By merely having faith in Jesus, you acknowledge you have also received deliverance from trying to do God's will in your own strength, such as keeping the Old Testament Law of Moses, including the dietary laws. Those laws were established to teach people how to recognize sin. Keeping these rules and regulations could never permanently bridge the gap between man and God. Jesus took care of that, fulfilled the law, and set us free. Freedom from the law means we are no longer in bondage to it for purposes of being in right standing before God. But we do need the law to remind us it is impossible to obtain the benefits of life as God's children without his help. So don't blatantly ignore these Old Testament laws. They contain practical wisdom God imparted to mankind because he knew we'd need it. After all, we are still flesh. We don't "do right" all of the time and must constantly rely on God for help in every area of life.

> *Likewise, my brethren, you have undergone death as to the Law through the [crucified] body of Christ, so that now you many belong to Another, to Him Who was raised from the dead in order that we may bear fruit for God. When we were living in the flesh (mere physical lives), the sinful passions that were awakened and aroused up by [what] the Law [makes sin] were constantly operating in our natural powers (in our bodily organs, in the sensitive appetites and wills of the flesh), so that we bore fruit for death. But now we are discharged from the Law and have terminated all intercourse with it, having died to what once restrained and held us captive. So now we serve not under [obedience to] the old code of written regulations, but [under obedience to the promptings] of the Spirit in newness [of life].*
> *~ Romans 7:4-6 (AMP)*

Watchman Nee, author of *The Normal Christian Life,* explains this truth perfectly. "It is God which worketh in you. Deliverance from law does not mean we are free from doing the will of God. It certainly does not mean we are to be lawless. Very much the reverse! What it does mean, however, is we are free from doing that will as of ourselves. Being fully persuaded we cannot do it, we cease trying to please God from the ground of the old man."

God is pleased when you admit you cannot function without him and you are relying on him daily. He wants you to include him in every area of your personal life — even when it comes to the contents of your refrigerator!

> *For by the death He died, He died to sin [ending His relation to it] once for all; and the life that He lives, He is living to God [in unbroken fellowship with Him]. Even so consider yourselves also dead to sin and your relation to it*

broken, but alive to God [living in unbroken fellowship with Him] in Christ Jesus. Let not sin therefore rule as king in your mortal [short-lived, perishable] bodies, to make you yield to its cravings and be subject to its lusts and evil passions. Do not continue offering or yielding your bodily members [and faculties] to sin as instruments (tools) of wickedness. But offer and yield yourselves to God as though you have been raised from the dead to [perpetual] life, and your bodily members [and faculties] to God, presenting them as implements of righteousness. For sin shall not [any longer] exert dominion over you, since now you are not under Law [as slaves], but under grace [as subjects of God's favor and mercy]. ~ Romans 6:10-14 (AMP)

So where do you go from here? I would say you should rejoice! Why? Because you are free! You are free from the guilt, condemnation, harassment, and sometimes embarrassment that come with recognizing you have not been a good steward over your temple.

Therefore, since we are justified (acquitted, declared righteous, and given a right standing with God) through faith, let us [grasp the fact that we] have [the peace of reconciliation to hold and to enjoy] peace with God through our Lord Jesus Christ (the Messiah, the Anointed One). Moreover [let us be full of joy now!] let us exult and triumph in our troubles and rejoice in our sufferings, knowing that pressure and affliction and hardship produce patient and unswerving endurance. And endurance (fortitude) develops maturity of character (approved faith and tried integrity). And character [of this sort] produces [the habit of] joyful and confident hope of eternal salvation. ~ Romans 5:1, 3-4 (AMP)

While you admit there is an area in your life that needs correction, you are not to endure the correcting process alone. If you have ever been to an Alcoholics Anonymous meeting or seen one portrayed on television, you will understand the point I (Kristy) am trying to make. All newcomers to AA must stand up and introduce themselves to the group and admit they are alcoholics. Next, the group welcomes the new guest and makes him feel at home. He is reassured he is in the right place to receive all the support and guidance necessary to conquer his addiction.

It should be apparent that as a Christian, you have one of the best resources available to help you turn your life around. This resource is so awesome that he is a doctor, a weight-loss specialist, a counselor, and a support system all rolled up into one. This Lord of health is also patient, so he will give you as much time and help as necessary to reach the full manifestation of your transformation. The book *Ministry of Healing: Health and Happiness* by Better Living Publications describes this reality best:

> Apart from divine power, no genuine reform can be effected. When one surrenders to Christ, the mind is brought under the control of the law; but it is the royal law, which proclaims liberty to every captive. Becoming one with Christ makes man free. Subjection to the will of Christ means restoration to perfect manhood. Obedience to God is liberty from the thralldom of sin, deliverance from human passion and impulse.

Hence, a true relationship with the Father is critical to conquering the flesh. There is no diet, doctor, hypnotist, or life coach who can lead you to the path of true health where you have the ability to resist the temptations of the enemy that may come disguised as an Oreo Double Stuff or a Whopper with extra bacon and cheese. I (Kristy) have been asked on numerous occasions how I am able to pass by fast food restaurants without being tempted to go in. My response has always been that I have learned how my body is made and what foods God has designated best for me to eat.

Without first committing my life to Christ and confessing Jesus as Lord of my life, I (Kristy) don't think I ever would have been able to view food the way I do now. The understanding I have regarding food selections and my health came directly from God. He has given me a new life, a new spirit, and internal power to resist foods I know could harm me. "And I will put my Spirit within you and cause you to walk in My statutes, and you shall heed my ordinances and do them" (Ezekiel 36:27 AMPLIFIED). And when I do occasionally eat something sweet and out of the ordinary, this new spirit also allows me to view the item as a treat and enjoy it, free of guilt and shame.

You may wonder why God would do so much for you. It is all because of his never-ending love for you. You are on his mind each and every day. God thinks about you all the time. He is saddened when he sees you suffering. Yet, he rejoices when he sees you succeed. God wants you to win the war on health. He desires that you have a fully functioning temple to carry out his specific assignment for you. He wants everyone to become a part of the body of Christ and bear fruit for the kingdom.

However, God knows our ability to focus on his work can be hindered by our own personal hang-ups. Whether you believe you are too fat, too tall, too short, or too small, God is accepting of you. He loves you for exactly who you are and only wants to see you become the best you can be in this lifetime. He understands you are going to make mistakes and does not expect perfection. He just asks that you acknowledge and remember all Christ acquired for you by going to the cross. Not only did you receive eternal life in heaven, you also received a guilt-free life here on earth.

So, make today the day you stop trying the latest and greatest diet program advertised on television, in magazines, and elsewhere. Stop aimlessly counting calories on the boxes of frozen cheesecake and cookies you routinely throw into your weekly grocery cart. Stop letting your unused two-year membership at the health club go to waste. Admit you need help in getting a grip on your health and run like a wide receiver to your heavenly Father. He is waiting to take you from the battlefield of defeat to a grace-filled victory party celebrating your new lifestyle of divine health.

> *Therefore, [there is] now no condemnation (no adjudging guilty of wrong) for those who are in Christ Jesus, who live [and] walk not after the dictates of the flesh, but after the dictates of the Spirit. ~ Romans 8:1 (AMP)*

Chapter Summary

1. God loves you and wants to help you to win this war on health.
2. The best way to conquer dietary strongholds is to first establish a relationship with God.
3. God's grace is always available to cover your mistakes — even when you fail to eat healthfully.
4. Jesus' crucifixion frees us from all guilt, condemnation, harassment, and embarrassment we may feel for not taking better care of our temples.

Chapter Twenty-Two

Sweet Surrender

But thanks be to God, Who in Christ always leads us in triumph [as trophies of Christ's victory] and through us spreads and makes evident the fragrance of the knowledge of God everywhere. ~ 2 Corinthians 2:14 (AMP)

A war ends when one side surrenders or defeats the opponent. But the struggle for divine health is different. It requires that you surrender *and* overcome the enemy. When you surrender to God's divine health plan you become empowered to keep Satan, who wants to kill you, under your feet. One of the definitions of "surrender" is "to give oneself over to something (as an influence or course of action); the action of yielding one's person or giving up the possession of something into the power of another" (*Webster's New Collegiate Dictionary*, 1981).

In the world system, surrender has a negative meaning. It teaches that the best life is one in which we do not surrender but instead push hard to get whatever we want and refuse to give up anything we hold near and dear. On this natural level, "surrender" often suggests weakness, defeat, or cowardice. But God's kingdom is a kingdom of opposites. Surrender in his kingdom means power, victory, and courage because we surrender only to him. We give up something that's not good to gain God's best. We give up lying for truth, strife for peace, taking for giving, unbelief for faith, complaining for praying, and weeping for laughing, and we replace many other burdens with the benefits of life as one of God's children. We even sing songs about it in church:

> I surrender all. I surrender all. All to Jesus, I surrender, I surrender all. (Judson W. Van de Venter & Winfield S. Weeden, "I Surrender All", chorus)

Perhaps many of you reading this book remember walking down a church aisle while the congregation sang this song. You met a pastor or elder, prayed the prayer of salvation, and accepted Jesus as your Lord and Savior. But did you really "surrender *all*"? True surrender is about an honest decision to change, and then your behavior eventually follows that decision. "All" means "all." It means not only giving up anger, unforgiveness, bitterness, carnal sins, etc., but also giving up physically unhealthy lifestyles. Your choice is clear. Give it up or give Satan license to kill you. Author Francis Frangipane, puts it this way in his book *The Three Battlegrounds*:

> Any area of our heart or mind not surrendered to Jesus Christ is an area vulnerable to satanic attack. And it is here, uniquely in the uncrucified thought-life of the believer's mind that the pulling down of strongholds is of vital importance. For this reason, we must attain what the Scriptures call 'humility of mind' before real deliverance is possible. When we discover rebellion toward God within us, we must not defend or excuse ourselves. Rather, we must humble our hearts and repent, exercising our faith in God to change us.

Isn't it wonderful that surrender is a choice God gives us that is birthed through faith and carried out through discipline? At face value, choice and discipline seem to be opposites. But the Apostle Paul describes how we should reconcile these principles so they work together for our good. In 1 Corinthians 10:23, he said: "All things are legitimate [permissible — and we are free to do anything we please], but not all things are helpful (expedient, profitable, wholesome). All things are legitimate, but not all things are constructive (to character) and edifying [to spiritual life]" (AMPLIFIED).

There is no law that tells us not to eat pancakes swimming in butter every day, but the fact that we are free to do so does not mean we should. The choice we make is actually a test of our character. "Character," as defined by *Webster's New Collegiate Dictionary*, is "moral excellence and firmness; the complex of mental and ethical traits marking and often individualizing a person, group, or nation." Character is shaped by our habits, actions, decisions, and thoughts. In order to have great character, these four areas must first be brought to a level of greatness. If we apply principles of great character to our health, we will show the world evidence of God's desire that we prosper and be in health even as our souls prosper. What will they see? They will see people who have the mind of Christ, walking around in the body Christ would want us to have, doing the things Christ would want us to do on earth.

One of the greatest nations in history got that way through discipline and lost its greatness due to the lack of it. Author Shannon E. French, in *The Code of the Warrior,* quotes Jewish historian Flavius Josephus in describing ancient Rome's renowned army:

> All their duties are performed with the same discipline, the same safety precautions: gathering wood, securing food if supplies were low, hauling water — all these are done in turn by each unit. Nor does each man eat breakfast or dinner whenever he feels like it; they all ate together. Trumpets signal the hours for sleep, guard duty, and waking. Nothing is done except by command. ... Absolute obedience to the officers creates an army which is well behaved in peacetime and which moves as a single body when in battle.

Will Durant in *Caesar and Christ*, the third volume in his series on civilization, notes the following about the Roman military:

> The major element in the success of this army was discipline. The young Roman was educated for war from his childhood; he studied the military art above all others, and spent ten formative years of his life in field or camp. ... Food in camp was simple: bread or porridge, some vegetables, sour wine, rarely flesh; the Roman army conquered the world on a vegetarian diet; Caesar's troops complained when corn ran out and they had to eat meat.

So for the Roman soldier, food was a resource – not a form of recreation. In stark contrast, upper class Romans satisfied their every appetite at mealtime. Durant says:

> Eating was now the chief occupation of upper-class Rome; there was in the ethics of Metrodorus, "everything good had reference to the belly." At a repast given in 63 by a high priest, and attended incongruously by Vestal Virgins and Caesar, the hors d'oeuvres consisted of mussels, spondyles, fieldfares with asparagus, fattened fowls, oyster pastries, sea

nettles, ribs of roe, purple shellfish, and songbirds. Then came the dinner — sows' udders, boar's head, fish, duck, teals, hares, fowl, pastries, and sweets.

Such indulgences by the Roman citizenry extended beyond mealtime. They were insatiable when it came to power, entertainment, etc. Needless to say, discipline and moderation were hard to find in the days before that once great empire fell. So this nation, including its remarkable army known for conquering rather than surrendering, imploded from within.

The body of Christ is God's military in the earth. In 1996, I (Christine) saw an amazing scene that seemed to exemplify or illustrate this role. Some would say I was dreaming, or in the body of Christ some of us might call it a vision. In any case, it was vivid and memorable.

For as far as I could see, there were soldiers dressed in army fatigues, standing in rank, and at full attention. There were too many to count. But this was no mediocre army. You could see their unity of purpose reflected in their eyes. Their gaze was steely — faces set like flint. They were sober and determined. As we would say today, they were all on the same page: fearless, fit, and extremely alert. No one moved. I'm not even sure they blinked.

The silence was even more compelling. You could have heard a feather drop in that stillness. The air was charged with anticipation. It was as if there was some kind of silent communion going on between them, although no one moved or spoke. There was a sense that what they were about to do would impact the whole world. This was no routine training mission. They were being sent straight into immediate battle. And the stakes were high.

The next thing I sensed, but never saw, was that these soldiers were facing their commanding officer. He was at the front of this massive group. I never heard him speak, but I sensed his presence all around. He was not a regular general or military officer. This leader was not subject to the whims of the Pentagon or the politics of the hour. He was fully in charge and was getting ready to take over something. Those who were with him were with him. And pity those who were against him. I felt this although I never saw his face.

Suddenly, I saw his arm extend and point to individual soldiers. When he did so, each soldier immediately fell out of rank and ran with clear purpose to a specific place to do a specific task. I do not know where they went but it was clear they knew where they were being sent, why they were going, and what they would do when they got there. No one debated about whether it was the right destination. They just went. Every time that pointing finger landed on a soldier, he or she took off running to comply with the silent order. Each went in different directions. I watched this in amazement for a while and then the scene faded away.

What did it all mean? Some will say nothing, that I had an odd dream, that we all have them and should not attach any particular meaning to these things. But I was so taken aback and frankly alarmed by the scene that I kept pondering it. I discussed it with a Christian friend and she, too, thought it had a meaning relevant to the body of Christ.

After a while, I sensed the following interpretation was on point: The soldiers were Christians. The commander in chief was the Lord God Almighty. The assignment related to work to be done by believers as we near the period of time the Bible refers to as "the last days" (see John 6:39 and 2 Timothy 3:1-9) or the end of the age. The pointing represented God's assignment to each believer — our marching orders to be carried out on earth — as well as the message that we need to get to them immediately.

Does the body of Christ today look more like this army or more like the citizens of the Roman Empire its latter days? Oh we talk the right talk. Conversations about spiritual warfare are often on our lips. We say things like, "Satan is bound. When he comes against me, I put him under my feet!" We quote Scripture, "No weapon formed against me shall prosper." And on and on we go with our religious speak. We also sing songs about being in God's army and on the battlefield for the Lord.

I (Christine) used to hear church folks sing enthusiastically about being a good Christian soldier when I was a kid. But in their lives away from church, they were getting slaughtered physically, mentally, and financially. Unfortunately, I still see some believers living this way and it must end. Are you truly battle ready or willing to get ready? Will you work hard to mature your spirit and prepare for war? Is your mind made up for Jesus and ready to follow his directions in the area of healthcare as well as everything else? Do you want your physical body in shape to serve as Jesus' hands and feet in the earth?

If the answer to these questions is yes, then the first order of business is to stop accepting sickness and disease as just the normal order of things. Kristy and I pray that a spirit of revelation — not condemnation — comes upon everyone reading this book. The spirit of shame and guilt must be bound. They are not of God, but are of the enemy and cannot produce any fruit, only more bondage. Satan wants people to feel so badly about how they have handled their health that they descend into hopelessness and make no effort to change. It is his age-old tactic.

Stop letting Satan convince you to live a life of excess and stop engaging in behaviors God either specifically prohibited or advised us to avoid. Don't let your past failures play like an audiotape in your head, over and over. And don't let the enemy kill off every instinct you might have to cry out to God for help, forgiveness, guidance, love, and comfort.

Do not apologize (except to God) for where you have been and where you are. Just decide to travel a different road that takes you back to the place of authority God gave us at creation. Chicago-area pastor Gregory Dickow once discussed the scope of this authority during a sermon. He said, "In order to walk in your full level of dominion and to have the ability to govern others, you must first learn to govern yourself. A hierarchy of government exists. Once you manage to govern yourself, then you are ready to govern your family. If you can govern your family, then you are ready to govern a village. If you can govern a village, then governing a city is possible. Lastly the ability to effectively govern a city, results in the ability to govern a country."

If you can't exercise dominion over something as small as a Twinkie, how can you exercise dominion over the work God has ordained for you to do? The simple answer is you cannot. And you also will not have credibility as God's ambassador on earth assigned to show the world a better way to live. But all of this can change. Yes! "Change," that dreaded word that seems to strike fear in many people, is critical to winning your fight to live.

Look in the mirror and ask yourself if you need to change your physical lifestyle in order to improve your health. If the answer is yes, ask God to show you what to do. He loves you and his intent is to preserve and not to punish. If God reveals to you that it is time to stop frequenting fast food restaurants, then you will have to make up your mind that you will stop and begin to carry your lunch to work. If he prompts you to get off the couch and start exercising at least three times a week, then whether or not you do it depends on the decision you have made to change your life.

To change literally means to take a different position, course, or direction. It also implies either making an essential difference, often amounting to a loss of original identity, or a substitution of one thing for another. Everybody has a need to change something about his or her life. God knew that after sin entered the world we would need help changing our course in order to get back to our rightful place in his kingdom. He is just waiting for us to enlist his divine assistance as we try to give up the things that undermine our walk with him.

So if you are continually feeling tired and sluggish, and your bouts with acid reflux and daily indigestion are becoming more than you can bear, something on the inside of you must decree that it is time to change your lifestyle. If you find yourself too tired to help your children with their homework or to keep up with their busy after-school schedules, then a change is long overdue. Your goal is to make a breakthrough in this area of life. So while deciding to skip the fries that come with your burger once is a good decision, it does not yield a breakthrough. Breakthroughs are the result of making good decisions multiple times.

Two keys to successful change are:

1. You must have a godly commitment to continual improvement. You must have a commitment that is not rooted in comparisons (leads to competition) (2 Corinthians 10:10) and a commitment that is not rooted in covetousness (greed). God has a purpose and a plan for us both individually and corporately. When you compare yourself to others, it takes you outside your assignment.

2. You must have a constructive discontent (Philippians 4). Don't be satisfied with the status quo. It is impossible to change if you are satisfied with the status quo.

Your desire for change must be pure. You can't decide to go on a temporary diet to lose weight just because your co-worker lost weight and has become the talk of the office. Neither can your decision to drop some pounds be based upon the desire to end your spouse's persistent nagging and complaints that you "need to lose weight." Your decision to improve your eating and thereby your health must be a personal decision that stems from the inside out and not from the outside in. The desire of your heart must be that you want to live for God and do everything possible to fulfill the purpose he has for you. Your goal must be to glorify God through both your spiritual *and* physical lifestyles. If your life is purpose-driven, then your food selections will be as well.

People want not only to *hear* about the benefits of life in Christ. They also want to *see* some fruit in the lives of those who proclaim his holy name and his plan for mankind. As God's walking, speaking spirit, the house in which you travel had better be up to snuff! Begin to see your physical well-being as an important asset to the kingdom of God that Satan wants to steal. Then fight to keep him at bay every time you are inclined to take the escalator instead of walking up a flight of stairs or every time you pick up a fork.

How do you do that on a practical level day after day? We're so glad you asked! A quick trip to your local bookstore will provide a wealth of resources with answers on how to manage your health from a practical standpoint. In our pursuit of healthy eating lifestyles, we have come across some good resources over the past few years. With love, compassion, and excitement, we share some of the information with you on the following pages. We also stand in agreement with you that you will receive revelation knowledge from the Holy Spirit about how to lead a healthier life that will greatly benefit the kingdom of God. Begin now to see yourself as an armed and dangerous soldier in the battle for your health and your divine destiny. And remember this instruction from I Corinthians 10:31: "Therefore, whether you eat or drink, or whatever you do, do all to the glory of God."

There are two obstacles to vibrant health and longevity: ignorance and complacency. ~ World Health Organization

Nutritional Education Resources

As authors, we have intentionally written this book to deliver a "why to eat healthy" message instead of a "how to eat healthy" message. Thus, we would like to suggest some resources that may help as you begin your journey towards divine health.

For an introductory seminar on the principles of "Fight to Live" and to spark a wellness revolution within your congregation or organization, contact:

Kingdom Come, LLC
Kristy Dotson & Christine Tennon
info@FightingToLive.com
www.FightingToLive.com

For in-depth nutrition education and "how to":

Nutrition Coach Network, LLC
info@NutritionCoachNetwork.com
www.NutritionCoachNetwork.com

Services include:
- Individual nutritional training (Virtual training available)
- Tours of health food stores with shopping tips
- Weight-loss programs
- Detoxification programs
- Nutrition deficiency testing & supplement recommendations
- Nutritional classes & workshops
- Corporate seminars
- Culinary classes

Additional Resources

Appleton, Nancy. *Lick the Sugar Habit*. New York: Avery. 1988.

Batmanghelidij, F. *Your Body's Many Cries for Water*. Falls Church, VA: Global Health Solutions. 1997.

Brownwell, Kelly, and Horgen, Katherine Battle. *Food Fight: The Inside Story of the Food Industry, America's Obesity Crisis, and What We Can Do About It*. New York: McGraw Hill. 2004.

Colbert, Don. *Toxic Relief*. Lake Mary, FL: Siloam. 2001.

Colbert, Don. *What Would Jesus Eat? The Ultimate Program for Eating Well, Feeling Great, and Living Longer*. Nashville: Thomas Nelson. 2002.

Colbert, Don. *What You Don't Know May Be Killing You*. Lake Mary, FL: Siloam. 2000.

Colbin, AnneMarie. *Food and Healing*. New York: Ballantine. 1986.

Cummins, Ronnie, and Lilliston, Ben. *Genetically Engineered Food: A Self-Defense Guide for Consumers*. New York: Marlowe. 2000.

Diamond, Harvey and Marilyn. *Fit for Life*. New York: Warner. 1985.

Diamond, Harvey and Marilyn. *Fit for Life II*. New York: Warner. 1987.

Fallon, Sally and Enig, Mary G. *The Cookbook that Challenges Politically Correct Nutrition and the Diet Dictocrats*. Warsaw, IN: NewTrends Publishing. 2000.

Fletcher, Kingsley A. *Prayer and Fasting*. New Kensington, PA: Whitaker House. 1992.

Gittleman, Ann Louise. *Fat Flush Plan*. New York, NY; Chicago, IL; San Francisco, CA; Lisbon, London, Madrid, Mexico City, Milan, New Delhi, San Juan, Seoul, Singapore, Sydney, Toronto: McGraw Hill. 2002.

Kadans, Joseph M. *Encyclopedia of Fruits, Vegetables, Nuts and Seeds for Healthful Living*. West Nyack, NY: Parker. 1973.

Kunjufu, Jawanza. *Satan, I'm Taking Back My Health*. Chicago: African American Images. 2000.

Lockman, Vic. *The Dietary Laws of the Bible*. Yreka, CA: Vic Lockman. 1997.

Malkmus, George. *Why Christians Get Sick*. Shippensburg, PA: Treasure House. 1989.

Mondoa, Emil. *Sugars That Heal: The New Healing Science of Glyconutrients*. New York: Ballantine. 2001.

Phillips, Bill. *Body for Life*. New York: HarperCollins. 1999.

Robbins, John. *Diet for a New America: How Your Food Choices Affect Your Health, Happiness, and the Future of Life on Earth*. Tiburon, CA: H J Kramer. 1987.

Rubin, Jordan. *The Maker's Diet*. Lake Mary, FL: Siloam. 2004.

Russell, Rex. *What the Bible Says About Healthy Living*. Ventura, CA: Regal. 1996.

Schlosser, Eric. *Fast Food Nation*. New York: Houghton Mifflin. 2002.

Stitt, Paul A. *Beating the Food Giants*. Manitowoc, WI: Natural Press. ISBN 0-939-956-06-6.

Walker, N.W. *Water Can Undermine Your Health*. Prescott, AZ: Norwalk. 1974.

Whang, Sang. *Reverse Aging*. Miami: JSP. 1990.

Woodford, Keith. *Devil in the Milk – Illness, Health, and the Politics of A1 and A2 Milk*. Nelson, New Zealand: Craig Potton Publishing. 2007.

CPSIA information can be obtained
at www.ICGtesting.com
Printed in the USA
FSOW04n1605311215
15102FS

9 780692 533741